ALL MY SECRETS

Messages of health from your body, decoded.

by
KUMARA SIDHARTHA MD, MPH
(With KAYLI ANDERSON MS, RDN, ACSM-EP, DipACLM)

Praise for Dr. Kumara Sidhartha's

All My Secrets: Messages of health from your body, decoded

" …Within each chapter is a treasure trove of knowledge explaining how the body works, what might make it go wrong, and, most importantly, steps to take to avoid that happening…"

- Kirkus Reviews

" With a story telling format, Dr. Sidhartha comprehensively captivates the good, the bad and the ugly of human physiology clarifying how it can injure and how it can repair every bodily system, simultaneously guiding you on the pathway to restore and maintain optimal health. "

- Caldwell B. Esselstyn, Jr., MD
Author *Prevent and Reverse Heart Disease*

"Internal medicine doctor Sidhartha debuts with a refreshing approach to understanding the intricacies of the human body. Sidhartha's approachable style makes the transition to a healthier lifestyle feel attainable for all readers, and he includes recipes at the end to help readers integrate his principles into everyday life, transforming healthy choices into sustainable habits. Readers wishing to take control of their health and pursue overall wellness will embrace this."

- Booklife Reviews by Publishers Weekly

"…Quite exceptional. Highly recommended for its educational content and writing style. ★★★★★ "

- Readers' Favorite

Copyright © 2024

Case ID #: 1-13560770343

eBook ISBN: 978-1-963609-82-0
Paperback ISBN: 978-1-963609-83-7
Hardback ISBN: 978-1-963609-84-4

All Rights Reserved. Any unauthorized reprint or use of this material is strictly prohibited. No part of this book may be reproduced or transmitted in any form or by any means, electronic or mechanical, including photocopying, recording, or by any information storage and retrieval system without express written permission from the author.

All reasonable attempts have been made to verify the accuracy of the information provided in this publication. Nevertheless, the author assumes no responsibility for any errors and/or omissions.

CONTENTS

ABOUT THE AUTHOR	I
ACKNOWLEDGMENTS	IV
DISCLAIMER	V
PREFACE	VII
CHAPTER 1. WITHERING ALLIANCE: EXCESS BODY WEIGHT	1
CHAPTER 2. TERROR WITH AN ACHILLES HEEL: CANCER	23
CHAPTER 3. UNPOPULAR RESISTANCE: DIABETES	43
CHAPTER 4. UNTANGLING THE GORDIAN KNOT: HEART HEALTH	64
CHAPTER 5. AGING: WHY THE RUSH TO AGE?	90
CHAPTER 6. THE SIXTH SENSE ORGAN: GUT FEELING	100
CHAPTER 7. IDENTITY CRISIS: AUTOIMMUNE DISEASES	118
CHAPTER 8. WORKING FRAME: JOINTS, BONES, AND MUSCLES.	132
CHAPTER 9. MEMORY SAVINGS FOR THE FUTURE: BRAIN HEALTH	159
CHAPTER 10. PRECIOUS MIRACLE: PREGNANCY	172
RECIPES	185
REFERENCES	265

ABOUT THE AUTHOR

Drawing from his 30 years of medical practice experience with a focus on nutrition, Dr. Kumara Sidhartha uses simple, everyday analogies and logic to break down the complex inner workings of the human body and the effect of food on these functions. Dr. Sidhartha completed Medical College at the Government Mohan Kumaramangalam Medical College in Salem, India, followed by Internal Medicine Residency training at Lincoln Medical Center, affiliated with Cornell University in New York. His pursuit of nutritional knowledge led him to complete a Master of Public Health in Nutrition at the University of Massachusetts, Amherst, Massachusetts. He is a contributing author in the textbook titled *Promoting Biodiversity in Food Systems* (1st edition, CRC Press, Taylor & Francis 2018). In 2016 he was the medical honoree of the American Cancer Society of New England for his efforts to prevent cancer through nutrition education of the community. He is board-certified by the American Board of Internal Medicine. He is certified in Plant-based Nutrition by e-Cornell University and T. Colin Campbell Center for Nutrition Studies. He currently practices internal medicine in southeastern Massachusetts.

https://kumarasidhartha.com

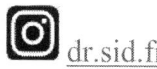 dr.sid.freshandwholesome

For Dad, for your generosity, compassion, and optimism.

We miss you.

For Mom, for your unconditional love and for showing grace and clarity of thought in the face of hardships.

ACKNOWLEDGMENTS

First and foremost, I want to thank my mom Rani Duraisamy and dad Dr. C. Duraisamy for ensuring me a safe and loving childhood which set the foundation for my life.

I want to thank my patients, both from India and in the United States. You entrusted your care to me and enriched my clinical career through your teachings. It has been my absolute honor.

In my journey to write this book, I was nudged, nurtured, challenged, cheered, guided, and motivated by family members and friends. I want to thank you all, for without your influence this book would not have made it over the finish line.

For a clinician like me, the self-publishing book world is an unfamiliar terrain. My sincere thanks to Lisa Thompson and Aiden Scott at Frontline Writers for your assistance in navigating this terrain to accomplish the procedural steps to publish this work.

I want to thank the many pioneers in the wholefood, plant-based medical discipline who blazed the path for others like me to validate the evidence behind the clinical benefits of this nutritional lifestyle. The list is too long for this page, however some notable giants of this field who explored this new frontier in recent decades include Dr. Dean Ornish, Dr. T. Colin Campbell, Dr. Caldwell Esselstyn Jr., Brenda Davis, RD, Dr. Neal Barnard, and Dr. Michael Greger.

I want to thank Kayli Anderson, Registered Dietitian Nutritionist, for her guidance with the recipes in this book.

DISCLAIMER

The information in this book is for general informational purposes only and is not intended as professional advice. The author and publisher make no representations or warranties regarding the accuracy or completeness of the information provided and will not be held liable for any errors or omissions. The opinions expressed in this book are those of the author and do not reflect the endorsement by or official policy or position of any agency, company or organization. Readers should seek professional advice as appropriate.

ALL MY SECRETS

MESSAGES OF HEALTH FROM YOUR BODY, DECODED

PREFACE

This is a story of secrets - about your body's inner workings. Secrets that I believe could add clarity to seeing your path to feel well and move with more energy while staying on that path. Sometimes, the mind could shift to the 'ignorance is bliss' mode and not want to dig in deeper. You may even be thinking, "Do I really want to know?" The truth is that the human body's default position is to heal and thrive well. To this end, it keeps sending signals to inform its likes and dislikes, hoping that we will pay attention and course-correct our behavior to maintain health and wellness. This communication between the body's inner workings and the person living in that body is fundamental to maintaining a healthy relationship with the body. As fundamental as open and honest communication is in any relationship. Your body yearns for you to be more attuned with it. One way to sync up with your body is by paying attention to its cues. And there are countless cues coming your way from the body every minute, even every second. One way to characterize this book is as a translator of these seemingly cryptic messages from the body to its person. Are you willing to tune in for a short while to unlock the body's secrets?

In this book, I hope to introduce you to the human body through the stories of nine individuals. Many of the characters are based on patients I have encountered in my nearly thirty years of clinical practice of medical and nutritional science, both in the Eastern and Western parts of the world. I have immense gratitude for what I have learned from these interactions along the way, which has shaped my understanding of how to be well.

The information shared in this book has varying levels of complexity. Wherever applicable, I have attempted to simplify using allegories and metaphors from everyday life. Each chapter will start with a synopsis in seven words and end with a summary of key points.

At this point, I would like to introduce you to your body to share some additional insights. To keep it simple, let me use a made-up nickname: Meet 'B,' your body!

B: Hello! This is fantastic. I am always looking to connect with the individual I am part of. I hope you stay tuned with me even after reading this book. Let me tell you a little bit about me before we get into the details.

I want to start by going back to the origins. The basics of how I came into being. It is not a hyperbole when people say the birth process is a miracle. Think about it. There are 64 trillion different combinations of genes that could happen between the 23 threads that carry genetic information ('chromosomes') from the man and 23 chromosomes from the woman during conception. One trillion is one million, millions! Not fifty million or five hundred million. One million, millions! Due to the sheer number of combinations that need to happen correctly and the principles of probability, there is a high likelihood of countless combinations that could deviate from the intended combination. Yet, I am born free of any such genetic deviations in 96% of conceptions. To put it in another way, there are 64 trillion combinations that could potentially diverge, resulting in an altered gene during conception. Let's first acknowledge that altered gene or not, every birth is a blessing in its own right. Altered genes can increase the risk of cancer, as seen in altered BRCA gene that protects against breast and ovarian cancer when not altered. On the flip side, some alterations come with beneficial effects, such as in Laron syndrome, where the individual is immune from getting cancer[1] due to an inability to produce insulin-like growth hormone-type 1 (IGF-1)[2]. In a later chapter of this book, I will share the inside information of Laron syndrome's immunity from cancer and how we can apply those learnings to prevent cancer.

Now, let's cut to the chase to allow me to tell you about something I have been wanting to tell you for a while. My likes!

I like to be nourished well, put to good sleep, create conditions that facilitate procreation to keep the genes going on to the next generations through the offspring, and I also enjoy sharing space with allies who protect me. These allies I am referring to are the 'good bacteria of the gut.'

Being nourished comes in many forms- not just food and water. It can be words, consuming positive information/news, or positive and healthy relationships. For starters, let's talk about food. I like nutritious food. The same way humans put higher grade fuel in their cars or juice from solar panels in today's electric car world, . Fresh, wholesome food. Mostly, they are rooted in soil and grow directly from the earth. It is frustrating to see that many modern foods hijack the feel-good system that I have in my brain that gives a sense of pleasure (*dopamine* system). But it comes with paying the price of damaging the car in the analogy (that would be damaging to me, the human body!). As the damage continues, when you and I have arthritis, cancer pain, or heart failure, the dopamine system is not stimulated to give a sense of pleasure but rather the signals of pain and discomfort that get fired up.

My next like: Adequate sleep is the equivalent of recharging the batteries of your phone or laptop in the night. I wish people would pay attention to recharging me (their bodies) with enough sleep as much as they recharge their devices. By the way, replacing the phone or laptop is easier than replacing the human body. I need more of this sleep when I am a baby and as I become an adult, 7 to 8 hours each night is just perfect. If I sleep way more than that when I am an adult, I am trying to send a signal that something is wrong.

Regarding carrying the genes through the offspring to the next generation, I motivate the person to procreate by rewarding the act by providing a sense of pleasure. I deploy my dopamine 'feel-good' hormone system for this reward.

I enjoy the company of healthy bacteria in my gut. When there is enough of the healthy ones, it is a story of a 'symbiotic' relationship where there is mutual benefit for both parties – that is, for me and the bacteria. It is the classic 'you scratch my back; I scratch your back' situation. So, what is in it for the healthy bacteria in this relationship? To put it simply, the undigested fiber in our meals serves as the 'meals' for healthy bacteria. To be more precise, the dietary fiber, as it goes through digestive processes, creates an environment that is conducive to the growth and sustenance of healthy bacteria. What do we, as the human host, get in return? A whole lot more that is out of proportion to what we give to the bacteria. The healthy bacteria are fundamental to governing how nutrients and calories are pulled out of the meals during digestion[3] as well as how the body can have a balanced immunity and avoid long-term inflammation. Considering the genetic material of the gut bacteria, it is very clear there are more of them than the native cells of the human body[4,5], enough to raise the question as to who is the host and who is the guest. More about this in detail later.

Now that I have shared what I like, let me share what makes me cringe and uncomfortable.

Not having enough hydration, excess or inadequate calories, meals that don't have dietary fiber or nutrients, being in 'fright-flight-fight' mode often, and exposure to things such as stress or unhealthy food make my daily wear and tear worse.

All these likes and dislikes are driven by a deep-seated set of goals, which I can share here:

Balance:

First and foremost, I like everything in my inner workings kept stable and balanced between the push/pull, the yin/yang, or whatever you want to call that magical place where two opposing forces co-exist in harmony and balance. An example is your blood sugar level. I aim to have the perfect balance between the insulin produced in your body to reduce excess blood sugar levels and the glucagon also made in your body but working to move your blood sugar in the opposite direction. When the push/pull effect of insulin/glucagon is in harmony, your blood sugar is maintained in perfect normal range, whether you miss a meal or not. This balance and stability is called *homeostasis* in science.

Homeo = similar or same; *Stasis* = stable,

Joy:

A state of bliss and comfort is a key goal of mine. I will let you know all about the dopamine system in one of the upcoming stories.

Avoiding harm that can come in the way of staying alive and healthy to propagate my genes through offspring to keep the species' genes going.

Spiritual inner-growth, whether one is religious, agnostic, or let's call it *getting wiser*, if you are an atheist: I, as the human body, am a transit vehicle for the person in it to learn from life's experience, evolve, and grow spiritually. In essence, the body can be seen as a train we get on for a journey of life-changing experiences that mature into inner growth.

Additionally, **realizing and reaching the full human potential** is another goal. Can you name a friend or a family member who has not realized his or her strengths? Most of you reading this can probably name someone before you finish reading this page. Hanuman is one of the most fascinating Hindu gods who illustrates the discovery of one's strengths and potential. Hanuman exemplifies empowerment, strength, loyal friendship, and excellent communication skills. All these elements are needed in our journey toward better health. In the Sanskrit epic *Ramayana*[6] from India, dating back to the 4th century BCE, Hanuman has the figure of part human and part monkey. He is a friend of the Rama, the prince of Ayodhya, and is considered as an avatar of the Hindu god Vishnu. The story goes like this: Prince Rama gets married to Seetha in an elaborate Indian wedding. Some unfortunate twists happen in the royal family's dynamics, due to which Rama gets instructions from his father, the powerful King Dasharatha. The command is for Rama and Seetha to live in exile in the jungle under challenging conditions for six months and to live in the royal court for the remaining six months of each year. Rama and Seetha leave for the wild jungle. When they try to navigate the jungle, Seetha gets abducted by the multi-headed demon King Ravana. She is taken to a remote island and kept imprisoned on a hill until she agrees to marry him. Rama is devastated when he realizes that Seetha is taken away. He tries to search for her and seeks assistance from his friend Hanuman. So, how does Hanuman teach about empowerment? When growing up, Hanuman didn't realize the enormous physical power he had due to a spell cast on him from his past. Not until he rescued Seetha from the dangerous territory of Ravana, did he know he had the strength to fly or lift up a mountain. In the setting of the necessity to help another person, Hanuman came to realize his powers when he was reminded of them by a saint who urged Hanuman to push beyond his comfort zone. When he tried to go beyond his comfort zone, Hanuman realized that he could actually do what he thought was impossible for him to do: rescue Seetha from the evil kingdom by flying across the ocean separating India and Sri Lanka, lifting the mountain off the face of the earth, and bringing Seetha back to safety. He literally moved mountains to achieve this. This Hanuman story teaches many of us that we have immense power that we don't realize until we push ourselves to the edge of our comfort zone and beyond. Whether it is a job you wanted to take up, a new skill you wanted to explore, a new food you wanted to try, or a new relationship you wanted to pursue - we all have the power to achieve that without realizing that we do. This mindset[7] is said to have the qualities of a person who has a lot of power but doesn't realize it. Another telling feature of Hanuman's efforts here is that he did something superhuman when it came to helping out someone else, not for helping himself. This, I think, goes to show a basic good quality of humans trying to go the extra mile when it comes to helping others rather than helping themselves.

Why does it matter in this book about healthy eating? I have come to realize that when I work with patients in facilitating their journey of eating healthy, they are more likely to stick to their long-term and short-terms goals of changing food habits if they do this for the benefit of someone else more so than doing it for themselves. For example, a grandfather who is contemplating improving his health by changing the food he eats is more likely to make that effort for the sake of living a healthy life in the coming decades to watch his granddaughter get married. This apparently is a more powerful incentive than making an effort to help his health. In our story, Hanuman pushes his limits when it comes to helping Rama, who is suffering from losing Seetha.

Hanuman's rescue efforts also speak to the loyalty of friendships. He did self-less acts that were superhuman in nature in order to help a friend who was suffering. Similarly, can one rise up to the challenge with acts of self-care when self-health is in danger?

As we saw in the friendship between Hanuman and Rama, having powerful, harmonious partnerships is helpful to get out of troublesome situations. In the first chapter, you will meet River and her potential allies. River, who has not realized her full potential like Hanuman once was and an army of trillions of defenders, waiting on the wings but withering due to uninhabitable conditions. What will it take for her dying army to survive and put up a strong defense? Let's find out in the next chapter.

CHAPTER ONE
WITHERING ALLIANCE: EXCESS BODY WEIGHT

> Seven-word synopsis
> **_Gut bacteria control weight through plant foods_**

The bright red streaks collided with the coffee-brown stripes as they came together as perfect swirls in the scoop on the spoon as it hit the tongue. Vanilla burst with sugar on the taste buds as the creamy texture coddled the brain, suspending all the senses somewhere between bliss and decadence. Cherry Mocha Vanilla is River's favorite ice cream. Little did River know that there were billions of tiny lives waiting in her intestines to rise up as an army of allies to help her out of this craving and to get her into a healthy relationship with her food. But all this army could do is wait until River makes the right move in her diet to set them in motion to help her out. More later on, what she could have done to fire up the allied army, but let's first meet River.

She is 30 years old. She, in her own mind, has "never been lovable." She also believed she had never been attractive either – well, at least that is what she was made to believe by all the movies, advertisements, conversations she watched growing up. River is in a bad place in her life because she works in a job that is unsatisfactory. Her second job is demanding-physically and emotionally. Her emotional state and not having a choice but to push 70 hours of work every week didn't leave much time to plan her life to take initiatives that could let her get ahead. She just came out of a bad relationship, and she keeps cursing herself for being born unlovable. "There is no chance of me becoming happy. I am *never* going to be in a happy relationship." River feels that her life isn't under her control. Not her job, not her relationships, not her two little kids. But her favorite brand of mocha chocolate ice cream *is* under her control. Every scoop of it. Nobody can stop her from that. River has struggled with her overweight issues for a very long time. Recently, it got worse. She hates the weighing scale. But she loves her friend Chandra, who is her high school buddy. Chandra is a twenty-two-year-old woman. River does feel blessed in certain areas of her life, especially the support system. She has had a great landlord for the past year, stabilizing her housing situation. She has a smart and wonderful accountant who has been making sure she doesn't make any missteps in her finance, given that her budget is tight. Above all, the core of her support system is through her friendship because Chandra is a gentle soul and wickedly funny. More importantly for River, Chandra is not someone who judges her. River feels she is so lucky to be around Chandra's supportive environment. I mean, who doesn't like laughter? And, who wouldn't love to be around people where you feel no judgment and you can be yourself totally?

    Chandra has roots in India, where her parents were born before moving to the United States. She grew up being exposed to the concepts of meditation and yoga. Having this cultural knowledge, Chandra has long nudged River to go for spiritual retreats, and finally, one day, River gets to sit for a meditation session during a weekend trip. During the session, she gets into a twilight zone where she was neither awake nor asleep. Most importantly, she didn't have the mental chatter that always kept saying negative things about her. In a surreal moment, she started seeing bright purple lights between her two eyebrows that gently slid and traveled to her neck. She started seeing the light move through a complex array of inter-connected cables, wires, and pipelines. She was beginning to sink into a subconscious state. She started a conversation with her own body.

River: Tell me a secret.

Body: I got lots. Which ones? Some can knock you down, and some can lift you up. How do you want to start?

R: Something that will knock me down. Let's save the good one for the end.

B: Well, for starters, you are not loving yourself deep down. If you love yourself, you will care for yourself better. The food you eat can be an indicator. How you nourish yourself tells how much you cherish yourself.

R: I don't know if I agree totally, but go on.

B: Your body and mind can get out of balance. See, everything in the body is kept in perfect harmony because of the balancing systems in place. For example, when you miss a meal and yet do physically demanding tasks, your sugar drops toward dangerous levels. Immediately, the human body responds with a shot of glucagon poured by the pancreas to bring up the sugar to safe levels. When the sugar is too much in the blood, a shot of insulin is poured into your blood by the pancreas to reduce the sugar to safer levels. See how perfectly the system balances the body. This is the balance that can be affected if we do things that repeatedly make this system work harder. It gives up this balancing act at some point, and the individual then develops diabetes.

R: Ok, but I don't need to get insulin injections for this, do I?

B: Well, let's see. You are overweight. Your last fasting blood sugar, when tested by her primary care physician, was 116. You are not yet there into the zone of definitive diabetes. Good news is that you can reverse it at this stage and bring your pancreas and sugar/insulin balance back to normal.

R: How? Does it mean I have to give up ice cream? I hope not.

B: The point here is you have the choice to take care of yourself at a deeper level. Choosing the other way hurts you slowly. What will you gain from reorienting your relationship with ice cream so that you control it rather than vice versa.

R: I don't know....don't I take care of myself by getting satisfied with a tasty scoop of ice cream? Why is pampering me with ice cream not equal to taking care of myself?

B: Well, you could see it as short-term gains or long-term gains. The sweet taste of ice cream is the short-term gain through the sense of getting pampered. Rebuilding your pancreas to function normally through better nourishment is the long-term gain.

R: This is all too deep. I have to think about it.

B: I know. It is a lot. While you are thinking about it, I would like to make this known. You and I are one entity, but currently, we are out of balance. The inner landscape of my workings in you has a lot of well-balanced systems that would normally work with more precision than today's computers would dream to mimic. The changes in your body in the process of gaining weight throw these intricate inner workings into disarray. This is making it harder to lose weight—kind of a vicious cycle.

R: Why is it so difficult for me to stop eating the bad stuff? I mean, I know that I should not be drinking that Frappucino or eating that hamburger with a side of French fries, but I can't stop it!

B: Well, before you think about beating yourself up for it, let me explain why you find it hard to control the eating. There is more than one issue that is working against you: the external factors, food factors, and physiological factors inside the body.

Let's first talk about some external factors that are outside of ourselves. The unhealthy foods are easy to buy. You don't have to drive miles and miles to get to them. And once you reach the store, they are right in front of you, at your eye level[8], so you won't miss it. And once your attention is now easily on this unhealthy choice, then it is a matter of making sure that price isn't a deterring factor to stop you from loading it into your shopping cart. So, cheap, unhealthy ingredients make for cheap, unhealthy food available for a dollar, more or less. The way the system works allows you to be around these foods easily and to make them affordable. Those are the exterior factors that shape the repeated behavior of bringing home things that you know you shouldn't be eating.

Let's look at food factors first. The manufacturers of foods that are processed and produced in a plant work extremely hard to ensure we don't stop with one chip from a chips packet, a cookie, or French fries. This process has been perfected as a science – literally. There are standards for designing and implementing such food science-related research and development. Millions of dollars are spent on meticulously developing the texture of the food, the feel of that food in our mouth, and the flavor mix that will leave our brain wanting more of that food and some more.

The perfect combination of sugar, salt, and saturated fat makes the brain feel pleasure and a bit of confusion, leading to wanting more of that food[9].

Another vital piece is our body's function and response to these foods. This is something very personal for me. As the human body, my workings involve not only structural entities such as the liver or heart but also other mechanisms through hormones that convey messages to different systems and parts within me. There are many hormone messengers that I use daily. There is a special set of hormones that come into play with regard to your issue of not being able to stop eating unhealthy food. The gut hormones.

R: Never heard of them. Should I presume that they are secreted by the gut?

B: Yes, for the most part. They are produced in the body from fat cells, the intestines, and part of the pancreas. These hormones can have a great deal of control over appetite[10] and related behavior through their actions on certain parts of the brain that regulate appetite, pleasure sensation, cravings, and addiction - namely the hypothalamus and the brain stem.

Let's talk about Leptin first. It is our 'off-switch' to stop eating. It decreases appetite and is the naturally occurring appetite suppressant we all are born with. It is secreted by the fat cells but works directly at the hypothalamus area of the brain to regulate appetite through two other chemical messengers in the body: neuropeptide Y and melanocortin[11].

As a person starts to gain weight, it has been shown that the Leptin levels start to increase to try and dam the appetite[12] and the calories coming into the body. However, it appears that in someone who is overweight or obese, the effect of Leptin to stop the appetite fails – an undesirable change called "Leptin resistance."[13] This is remarkably similar to the 'insulin resistance.' The latter is believed to be the main reason why people get diabetes. In such individuals with 'insulin resistance,' their own natural protection to control blood sugar, through insulin from their pancreas, doesn't work well in the obese setting. Similarly, Leptin, a natural protection against craving, doesn't work well in the obese setting due to 'leptin resistance.'

R: What goes wrong with the Leptin?

B: As I mentioned, the Leptin signals don't work in the brain area called the Hypothalamus. This results in failure to send the "I am full- I can-stop- eating-now" signal from the brain. This failure is directly related to regular consumption of diets high in fat, sugar and low in fiber[14, 15], resulting in the lack of having a strong barrier ("mucosal layer[16]") in the lining of the gut and elevated blood cholesterol levels such as triglycerides[17]. It is notable that in this lining, there is a mix of immune cells, messengers, and bacteria -both harmful and beneficial ones. We all have a mix of the good and bad bacteria, but it is a question of which one is dominant in numbers that determines a whole lot of our health. This barrier[18] in the lining of the gut is what is standing in defense between harmful bacteria and our bloodstream in the deeper layers of the gut lining. A breakdown of this barrier can result in the wall becoming fragile and leaky[19, 20]. Harmful bacterial elements gain entry through the gaps in the protective wall and create a toxic state in the system, medically called 'metabolic endotoxemia[21].' The result of this toxic state is that the leptin signals fail to launch the 'off-switch' from the brain to help us stop eating during a meal. This is one of those situations where the attacking bacteria that enter the system through the break in the gut lining wall didn't have to breach the wall themselves but only had to wait for the wall to be breached through meals that are high in fat and sugar and low in dietary fiber[22, 23]. The person consuming these foods through habit, culture, and lack of information and opportunity to explore other foods will unknowingly just go through slow self-destruction of his/her own gut's defense.

On the other hand, a healthy meal pattern that is high in fiber and low in fat and sugar is associated with a high diversity of the good, beneficial bacteria in the lining of the gut, including an abundance of species involved in stimulating mucus production which builds a strong defense barrier in the gut[24]. The combination of an intact mucus layer and tight intestinal lining with no gaps results in an intact gut barrier that keeps the brain's signals flowing normally to regulate appetite[25] through its 'on' and 'off' switches turned on and off appropriately.

Cholecystokinin (CCK)[26], another hormone secreted by our small intestine, sends the signal to the brain that we are full from the meal, thus helping to stop eating.

R: Okay. Didn't you say that you have something you say that will lift me up? I am ready.

B: Surely. Amazing things can happen when you take care of the body by nourishing it with a little bit of care. My systems always want to repair on their own and get back to working condition so the machinery of the body can keep working. I have stuff in each cell ready to repair when things break down. More importantly, I have an army of allies and cheerleaders waiting to help us maintain a normal body weight. An army that is many billions plus strong in numbers.

R: Which army?

B: Say hello to our little friendly bacteria buddies in our gut. There are countless bacteria in our intestines collectively called 'microbiome.' There are basically two types: the good ones and the bad ones. The friendly 'good bacteria' need us, and we (you and I) need them, especially if we want to avoid long-term diseases, under-prepared immune defenses, food addiction, or excess weight problems. These little minions are working in our best interests to create a healthy inner environment in the gut through their interactions with the right food in the gut. Especially food with dietary fiber, such as legumes, beans, greens, vegetables, fruit, and whole grains. The healthy bacteria, in order to thrive, need dietary fiber. When these bacteria breakdown the fiber in our diet to release a type of fatty acid called Short-Chain Fatty Acid (SCFA)[27]. Many favorable signals in the body are triggered by the action of these SCFAs[28]. One such is how these fatty acids stimulate our gut hormone factories to produce more of the hormones that rein in our appetite[29]. These appetite-suppressing hormones are called Glucagon-like Peptide-1 (GLP-1) and Peptide YY. These SCFAs also suppress excess appetite through another mechanism. Joining their little 'hands' with our dietary fiber, they work as a team to slow the release of craving-inducing ghrelin, a hormone secreted mostly by the stomach and, to a lesser degree, by the small intestine. These gut hormones stimulate appetite and cravings by working on the brain's reward and pleasure headquarters that govern food cravings, addiction, etc.

R: Little minions that have far-reaching effects at the control tower in our brain!

B: Exactly! Gut bacteria (good and bad) and their genetic material are collectively called the 'Microbiome.' The chain of events and coordination between the brain-gut-microbiome (BGM)[30] works with precision - as long as we are eating dietary fiber in our meals. One of the best foods that produces high amounts of beneficial SCFAs by bacterial fermentation in the gut is beans/legumes[31]. Supplying beans[32, 33] to our gut pays off with returns in the form of SCFAs[34] that protect the colon from cancers, reduce food cravings, regulate appetite, govern how much calories are absorbed,[35] avoid excess body weight, prevent allergies[36], and reduce long-term inflammation, which in turn reduces risk for long term diseases such as heart disease, diabetes, cancer, auto-immune diseases, and allergies.

You may recall we talked about 'homeostasis', the balance between opposing functions in the human body that, when kept in the right balance, governs pretty much everything about ideal health in the human body. The same goes for the balancing act between the forces that increase appetite and craving and the forces that keep them in check. What is on our menu for the day (hint: dietary fiber) determines how effectively the beneficial bacteria can maintain this balance to govern a majority of the levers of long-term good health.

R: I better start feeding my allied army by eating more meals with dietary fiber. I wish I knew this sooner. I should have started working on this when I was younger.

B: Well, you did the best you could with what you knew and the situation you were in. The positive news here is that you are now aware of why you are struggling with your meals and health and how you can start to get out of this. I know that your life has been stressful, with many stressors coming your way in the past few years. Dealing with that long-term stress wasn't easy for you because you didn't have coping skills and tools for resilience to deal with stressful life situations. That would have made it harder for you to try out changing your diet during that time. In fact, it would be much easier to deal with cravings if we had developed coping skills to deal with stress.

R: How is that connected to food cravings? Give me an example of a coping skill.

B: Well, the mindfulness meditation you are trying now is an example of a coping skill to deal with stress. To learn how long-term stress is connected to eating habits[37], let's re-visit the messenger of bliss from food - the dopamine molecule. First, we need to understand what happens when the human body is exposed to long-term stress that leaves the body exposed to 'flight' 'fright' or 'fight' mode of living for many hours during the awake hours.

During such time, the higher hormonal control center in the brain called 'the hypothalamus' releases 'supervising' hormones that work on the hormone-secreting gland next to the kidney called 'the adrenal' glands to release hormones that allow the person to handle sudden danger. Hormones of natural steroids are released from the adrenal glands at more than normal levels. These excess steroids ('glucocorticoids') have a blunting effect on the ability of the gut-brain circuit[38, 39, 40] to effectively convey the pleasure signal to the brain for foods that have high sugar, high fats, or high salt.

R: Give me an example.

B: Let's say you have a friend who is eating foods high in fats or sugar or salt. On top of that, life is stressful for that person. And, you, the individual, also don't have coping skills to deal with the stressors. That's a perfect storm. For the same level of high fat, high sugar, or high salt food that person was enjoying the pleasure of eating, now the taste buds are unable to convey the final message of pleasure. This is due to excess levels of corticosteroids that come in the way of the communication circuit that stops the bliss message from reaching the brain cells that need to make the person feel satisfied with that meal. They do this by taking down many docking stations in the brain[41] that are designed specifically to receive the incoming dopamine molecules that carry the 'I am-in-bliss' message.

R: Well, it appears that I am on the right track with not only learning about eating but also with the learning of coping skills such as mindfulness meditation. I know I need to make some changes in my eating, but I have always felt like I am stuck.

B: Can you tell me more about it?

R: Status quo in my eating is a happy place to be, and when I try to change my eating to something healthy, it tastes like cardboard. I can't eat cardboard all my life.

B: How do you know that is the case where the taste of healthier foods will remain like cardboard for life?

R: I don't know. I guess I am assuming that.

B: It is not life long but rather 2 or 3 months for the taste buds to reset the threshold for sending the pleasure signal to the brain for tasty, healthy food. No more cardboard after that, even when eating healthy meals.

R: How does that work?

B: When we get introduced to foods with an excess of salt, fat, and sugar, our taste buds get 'spoiled' and expect that abnormally high level concentration of sweets, salt, and fats to fire the happy signal to the brain. This is an altered brain signaling pattern that is not normal[42]. This introduction to such unhealthy food choices could happen as a kid or even as an adult. With this habituation, the 'reward' centers in your brain are expecting more of the high fat, high sugar to make you feel the pleasure from the food. No level of excessive sugar, salt, and fat is too high. And that is abnormal. A regular strawberry or a carrot can't stand a chance in this setting unless you give it a few weeks for the signaling system to reset in order to have a juicy strawberry feel like a satisfactory treat.

R: That explains my multiple failed attempts to change my meals to healthy food. I would try to eat better, and as soon as I feel that 'cardboard,' I would revert back to the usual diet that kept me in a satisfied place.

B: That makes sense. You go back to eating high-fat, high-sugar, high-salt meals. It serves the tongue as the master in this abnormal relationship with your food. This servitude to the tongue happens at the expense of other vital organs of the body. That is why you are stuck in a vicious cycle that keeps you tethered in this dysfunctional relationship with food that is more harmful than beneficial. You end up in a continuous loop of cravings, abnormal brain signals related to appetite control, and a sense of pleasure from food, and inflammation in the body and brain.

R: What is inflammation?

B: If you bump into a table, your arm can develop a contusion with swelling and pain. A defense army of white blood cells arrives in that location to clean up dead cells following that injury. They also defend against any attempts by bacteria on the skin trying to enter through the broken skin. This reaction is inflammation. Same thing when it happens in the bronchial tubes in the lungs is called bronchitis. Usually, it is a short-lived event, and it has a purpose to defend and clean up after an abrupt event. But when this inflammation becomes long-term for years in response to daily insults in the form of unhealthy breakfast, lunch, dinner, and snacks in between, then it becomes an abnormal state of the human body. Most of the long-term diseases of today are a result of this long-term inflammation, including cancers, diabetes, heart attack, stroke, dementia, auto-immune diseases, stroke, inflammatory bowel diseases, etc.

R: I can't believe I got stuck on this craving cycle that I can't get out. How did I get here?

B: Lack of dietary fiber and addition of excess fats and sugars altered your gut microbiome, changing the brain's appetite regulation. This started having more appetite for bigger portions as well as cravings for higher fat/sugar food and snacks in order to feel pleasure from food. The excess calories you consume are packed away as 'visceral fat' deep inside your abdomen, close to your intestines. This 'visceral fat' is like a factory of inflammation-provoking molecules[43] that would keep me in a constant state of inflammation.

Your brain gets bathed in this inflammation that messes with the control center for the reward system that normally sends dopamine messengers to feel bliss for the right amount and types of food. Due to the effect of this 'neuro-inflammation[44, 45]' two things go wrong:

1. Cravings increase because the brain expects more of the unhealthy food to make the person feel pleasure. Hint: this is the same process in any addiction, whether it is food, alcohol, or gambling.

2. The other effect of neuro-inflammation is that it makes the 'appetite turn-off' switch work less effectively.

This, in turn, results in less consumption of food that is high in dietary fiber that doesn't taste as good as your favorite foods. Without a steady inflow of this dietary fiber, the beneficial bacteria waiting in your gut are starved[46] and exposed to an environment that is not viable. Remember what happened to Napoleon's army when his soldiers were made to march in the severe winter of Russia. Your army of friendly bacteria is tested in the same way based on what's on your menu for the day. Adding more dietary fiber in the meals feeds this army in your gut to defend you better. I hope that lifts you up, knowing that help is waiting on the wings to get you out of this place of dysfunctional relationship with food that you have been stuck in for many years.

R: I am ready. I need to get off this craving cycle.

B: Yes, the sooner, the better because your eating choices are creating the early stage of diabetes. The stage is called pre-diabetes and is totally connected to inflammation and visceral fat. The inflammation happens all over your body when you are eating your favorite ice cream. It happens subtly and sneakily so you don't feel it, unlike how you would feel that inflammation after bumping into a table.

R: Can I do something about it? Should I be taking an anti-inflammatory medication for this?

B: Yes, you can do something about it. Taking anti-inflammatory medications is an incomplete approach.

R: Why do you call it incomplete?

B: Treating inflammation doesn't address the problem of why inflammation happened in the first place; it doesn't address the root cause of the problem. In scientific lingo, it is called a "reductionist" approach.

R: I am not getting it. Give me an example.

B: I will give you a story. Do you know about the story of few blind men and the Elephant?

R: No, tell me about it.

B: In a remote village in Asia, a few blind men in the village get curious to know what an elephant looks like, so they come up with a plan to figure this out. They go to the temple with an elephant statue, and each one of them touches the elephant to get a sense of what an elephant looks like. The man who touched the elephant's tail screams, "An elephant looks like a rope!" "No, an elephant looks like a snake," screams another man who got very fearful after touching the moving trunk. Another guy, who touched the tusk, visualized an elephant looking like a spear. And so on. The problem with these blind men was that they couldn't see the whole picture. Due to their limited perception, they were imagined. This is the same reductionist problem in viewing health and chronic diseases. If we don't see that inflammation is part of a whole sequence of changes with common root causes of poor nutrition, then we will be targeting each individual problem with individual solutions. That is how I end up having to deal with the a separate pill an individual takes for diabetes, a different pill for cholesterol, and another pill for arthritis when in fact, all these diseases have a common root cause of inflammation through poor dietary choices.

So, taking anti-inflammatories is a band-aid that addresses one part of the big problem in a very superficial way.

Two of my partners don't like being overworked, so I want to discourage you from taking anti-inflammatory medications for this. They are like a band-aid or worse than a band-aid. At least band-aids don't get into your system that much to challenge other organs, but anti-inflammatories do.

R: Which partners?

B: Your kidneys and your liver. They have to work hard to handle the anti-inflammatory medications that don't even address the root cause of the problem.

R: So if taking a pill to stop the inflammation is not the best option, then how do we go about it? Where is this inflammation originating so we can target that location?

B: The location where all the inflammation is in the brain and in our fat cells. To be more precise, it is the fat cells located deep inside the abdomen, right next to the intestines. It is called 'visceral fat.[47]' That is the factory where the molecules that bring forth inflammation are mass-produced and released into the system. The bigger the mass of visceral fat, the more inflammatory molecules are released into the system.

R: Is there a way to shrink the visceral fat?

B: Surely. It is all about the calorie balance or net calories between calories in and calories out. 'In' through food, 'out' through physical activity. So, when there is a negative balance, meaning fewer calories enter the body relative to the amount of calories burnt, the visceral fat starts to shrink. The reverse is true as well. When fewer calories are burnt or when there are excess calories consumed relative to the amount burnt, it has the same result - build-up of excess calories in the form of visceral fat.

Now, let's discuss how you can get off the cycle of cravings, inflammation, and more cravings.

Fundamentally, you need to start feeding and empowering the army of friendly bacteria to do the heavy lifting to reverse your cravings.

It won't be easy in the first 6 weeks to 6 months, when your taste buds rebel against this transition by making your new foods taste like cardboard, with the hopes that you will give up trying to change your meals. Can you hang in there for those weeks? Who will be your motivating support system when you are trying to embark on this change?

R: What do I need to stop these cravings?

B: Consider replacing high-fat meals with choices that introduce fiber with more vegetables, leafy greens, whole grains, and legumes for protein. Switch high-sugar snacks with fruit. This will start feeding the army of friendly bacteria that want to fight on your side.

Let's keep in mind that up until you start to change your meals, your taste buds are used to high concentrations of sugar, fat, and salt. Essentially, the threshold to have the brain feel pleasure from any food has been elevated[48] to such a degree that the taste buds scream "cardboard" when you introduce dietary fiber-rich foods with not as much sugar, salt, and fat. So, what should taste good, such as strawberries and carrots, now are perceived as 'cardboard'. The key is for you to know that it takes a few weeks to get the taste buds to not have such a high threshold to send the signal to the brain that the food is tasty. Over a period of 6 weeks to 6 months, gradually, the threshold will be reset. Then strawberries and dates feel like desserts.

R: Will this help to stop the craving cycle I am stuck in?

B: Yes. As your taste buds act normal, it will have you sense pleasure and satisfaction when eating healthy, wholesome foods rich in dietary fiber without much fats, salt, and sugar. These foods get the friendly bacteria in your intestines to regain their footing and start proliferating. They will produce more of the short chain fatty acid (SCFAs) as part of their interaction with the dietary fiber. These SCFAs help to reduce the local inflammation[49] in the gut lining. More importantly, they start rebuilding the fence to stop the harmful bacteria from getting through the fence and slip into the bloodstream to make the body toxic with inflammation. Without such intrusion and related inflammatory toxins messing up the brain's appetite control centers, your cravings start to come down to a halt while, at the same time, your appetite is more normally regulated by the 'off' and 'on' switch for the appetite.

R: That's hopeful. 6 months is too long to go through the transition.

B: Every month will be a better month after the first 2 months. Hanging in there for the first 2 months is the key.

R: Do I need to do a complete swap of all my meals? Hope not!

B: Not at all. Start replacing 2 meals every week and before you know it, in 2 months, you will discover 16 new meals for the weekly menu! Remember, we have 14 to 21 meals per week, depending on whether one eats 2 meals a day or 3.

Don't forget to get a friend or family member to be the check in person to motivate you to go through the transition in the first 2 months. Over the next 6 weeks, the change in the meals will start resetting the cravings, the appetite regulation, inflammation and anti-inflammation balance, all beginning to set the stage for moving toward ideal body weight and reducing the risk and impact of long-term inflammation. As the excess weight starts to drop, not only is the fire of inflammation being put down, but also the production of too much estrogen that increases the risk for breast cancer starts to go down.

R: Wait, what does the excess body weight have to do with estrogen and cancer?

B: Well, we usually associate estrogen production with ovaries as the source; however, in adults, the estrogen produced by ovaries starts to dry up while the fat cells in the excess fat begin to put out more estrogen into the bloodstream. This excess fat is from not having the optimal balance of caloric intake and burning of calories, leading to storage of excess calories as fat in the liver, visceral fat, and fat elsewhere in the body. When breast cells in a woman get bathed by this excess estrogen floating in the blood after overproduction in the excess fat cells, that sets the stage for breast cancer.

R: I didn't realize that excess body fat is a risk for breast cancer. I always thought that genetics and family heredity was the reason for breast cancer.

B: Well, over 90% of breast cancer out in the community are not determined by genetic defects carried over from one generation to the next. They are in a small yet significant percentage of cancers (under 10%)[50]. In a majority of the individuals with breast cancer, the genes have no defects at birth to increase risk for breast cancer but rather develop the problem after birth and can be avoided by modifying lifestyle.

R: Interesting! Tell me more about cancer.

B: I will. But before we go there, let's summarize the key points:

1. Microbiome rebuilds the gut's lining and orchestrate gut hormonal messenger communications between gut and brain to control appetite
2. Beans helps the friendly bacteria produce more of the short-chain fatty acids (butyrate) which releases and sustains GLP-1, the appetite-curbing molecule of popular weight loss drugs!
3. Leafy greens and other fiber-rich plant food such as vegetables, fruit and wholegrains feed the friendly bacteria with the necessary fiber to keep them strong; in return these bacteria keep us healthy.
4. Foods high in sugar and fats and low in dietary fiber result in Leptin resistance that breaks the appetite 'off-switch.' This triggers a loop of craving for these foods that turbo charges the craving further into uncontrollable levels.
5. Long-term stress can blunt the satisfying effect of high sugar and high fat foods resulting in excess consumption.
6. Inflammation, visceral fat and neuro-inflammation – impact appetite regulation and results in overconsumption and excess body weight.
7. Excess body fat releases excess estrogens, heightening breast cancer risk in women. Reducing excess body fat reduces risk to breast cancer.

CHAPTER TWO
TERROR WITH AN ACHILLES HEEL: CANCER

> Seven-word synopsis
> ***Plant foods block all common cancer paths***

Body (River's): Heard of Ms. Angelina Jolie, the actress?

R: Are you kidding? Of course, I have.

B: Then you may also know that Ms. Jolie had double mastectomy surgery[51]. What people may not know is that the genetic risk that individuals like Ms. Jolie are born with is linked to a breast cancer *protective gene* gone wrong due to a glitch at the time of conception. The BRCA gene is a protective gene that prevents breast cancer[52]. When I manifest in different people, I come with a package of protective traits in the cells – like the BRCA gene. In other words, at birth, I am a perfect design with built-in checks and balances that always protect YOU. It is very rare for the genetic glitches to happen during conception.

R: Then why do some people develop cancer while others don't?

B: With regard to individuals such as Ms. Jolie, being born with a BRCA gene mutation- a glitch in the gene, places them at higher risk of breast cancer because the built-in protective effect in the cell is lost with the glitch in the BRCA gene. *These instances of genetic defects happening at conception are very rare compared* *to genetic defects that happen as and when someone is growing up into adulthood.* For every genetic risk sealed during conception, thousands of genetic risks start AFTER the person is born and is growing up rather than at her/his birth. Nine out of ten cancers are not related to heredity or genes but rather due to glitches in the genes due to exposure to harmful elements (mostly through diet or harmful substances such as nicotine or alcohol) to a degree that overwhelms the in-built inherent compensatory protective mechanisms in us. The same is true for breast cancer. The bigger point here is that we can keep the protective genes safe by making healthy food choices and avoiding harmful food. This way, I can continue to do what I am best designed to do: protect you from diseases.

R: I get the broken gene concept you mentioned. I know it is rare for that to happen at birth. Only 1 out of 10 breast cancers are related to such birth defects in these cancer genes. How about the other 9? Are you saying food plays a significant role when cancer forms in the other 9 out of 10?

B: Great question. Cancer occurs when there is a perfect storm. For this perfect storm to build up, a few things need to come together in your body (i.e., me). I can explain this cancer process in two steps. ***Step one*** involves the initiation of cancer[53]. This is when cancer-inducing chemicals or viruses, commonly called 'carcinogens,' come into contact with the cells and their genetic material, called Deoxyribonucleic acid, known as DNA. It is this DNA that carries genetic information passed on from one generation to the next, as well as protective genes that guard against cancer. The carcinogens "initiate" the chain reaction that ultimately results in cancer by creating a lot of "free radicals" in the cells[54]. These "free radicals" are also called "oxidants" and cause a type of biological stress on the cells called 'oxidative stress.' If your cell is the China shop, then free radicals are the bulls. You know what happens when there are bulls in the China shop. Things get broken. Why do these free radicals behave like bulls in a China shop? They are looking for donors, and they are agitated.

R: Really? Are they looking for money??

B: Well, in this case, they are looking for a donor to donate an electron.

R: Go on.

B: These free radicals, at a molecular level, have electrons circling around in their structure. These electrons are usually in pairs. When they are single, they are trouble.

R: Well, I would have guessed that part.

B: That's right. When one of the electron's status is single and available it is agitated with extremely high energy and behaves unpredictably[55]. It becomes an unstable molecule and bounces around the cell knocking down important, fragile stuff in the body. One of these delicate China dishes in the shop is the nucleus of the cell with all the precious DNA material. If the bull population increases in the micro shops (our organs' cells), the China dishes fall victim to their rogue behavior. The DNA material in the genes inside the cells gets broken when too many of these high-energy free radicals are floating in the cells. Science calls it gene mutation. In our analogy, broken genes are broken China dishes. Because these genes are coding for protective processes in the body against cancer, these genes can no longer protect us from cancer when broken. Broken genes, if left unfixed, will increase the chances of cancer. How do we stop these bulls? By donating an electron. Once they get their electron to make the single electron paired, the bull snoozes. That is, the high-energy 'oxidant' molecule becomes more docile and stops posing a threat to the protective genes in our DNA.

R: Wow! How do we get donors for electrons?

B: Well, the donors are commonly called anti-oxidants[56]. They are found in the pigment that gives the color for colorful fruit and vegetables[57, 58]. Anti-oxidants are found in some herbs and spices[59].

R: Okay, I get it. I have to eat more colorful fruits and vegetables regularly to keep these bulls quiet so that they don't break the DNA material.

B: You got it.

R: Who fixes these broken genes if they get broken?

B: That is where I come in. As your body, I come equipped with a slew of fixing tools to prevent DNA breaks and to fix them when they happen[60]. I prevent the DNA breaks by reducing the power of the "bulls in the China shop." I can reduce the energy of the free radicals and make the bulls snooze. I do that by using protective anti-oxidants in the cells that work to slow down these oxidants. Of course, I depend upon the person to eat enough colorful fruit and vegetables to boost up the dose of protective anti-oxidants in the cells. The other way the person can prevent or minimize the DNA breaks is by limiting exposure to carcinogens such as tobacco, toxic chemicals, etc., by not using tobacco, and by reducing the toxic chemical load that enters the body.

R: You mean by choosing organic food?

B: More importantly, by eating at the lower end of the food chain. That is, eating mostly plants or plant-based food.

R: Explain. What happens at the higher end of the food chain that is of concern?

B: The toxic chemicals are found at the highest concentration in the flesh of the members at the top of the food chain. In other words, lions, sharks, and humans- all the top predators holding their space at the top of the food chain- end up with most of the toxins found at the bottom of the food chain. You may recall a health advisory regarding exposure to toxic levels of mercury for pregnant women. The advisory calls for avoiding the intake of certain types of predator fish, such as tuna or shark which are members at the top of the food chain. That is for exactly the same reason. So, let's look at this a bit more closely. Imagine a food chain that is depicted using a food pyramid with its peak pointed skyward. On the bottom, you have grass, plants, grains, etc. On the next level of the pyramid (narrower in width), you have the herbivores that eat the plants. Why is the next pyramid level narrow? Because 1000 units of plants at the bottom of the pyramid can support only 100 units of herbivores. Why is this? Because not all solar energy that enters the 1000 units of plants ends up in the next herbivore level. Some of the solar energy is wasted in this process of how energy moves up the food chain. This loss of energy is called "entropy." It is based on the second law of thermodynamics. It is physics.

R: It has been a long, long time since I read any physics. It was fun learning about the phenomenon of "gravity and the apple falling from the tree?"

B: Correct. You are referring to the Newton's law. What we are talking about are the laws of thermodynamics. Let me make it quite simple. Remember how you light up the headlamp in a bicycle by pedaling the cycle that moves a roll over the rim of the moving wheel to power the headlamp?

R: Yes, magical.

B: Well, that represents the first law of thermodynamics. Energy can neither be produced nor destroyed but rather transferred from one state to another. In the case of a bicycle, energy is transferred from the mechanical state of the spinning wheels to the electrical state, which lights up the headlamp. Here, the mechanical energy of the pedaling and the spinning wheels generate electrical power inside a coil of wire that holds a magnet which is then transferred to the headlamp. Now that we have the first law covered, let's move on to the second law of thermodynamics, which is directly related to why eating plant-based foods minimizes the carcinogen load to prevent cancer.

R: Go on.

B: Second law: The second law in the nutrition and cancer world may be renamed as the "law of going organic - the cheap and efficient way." You are going to see why I call it by this name. Energy always moves from a source of higher concentration to a lower concentration. The sun has the most energy, and the solar energy moves from the source of highest concentration (the sun) to the next level of plants. The leaves of plants take up solar energy to make starch using the process of photosynthesis. So, plants have the next (lower) amount of solar energy. Some of the energy from the sun is lost in this process. It is called entropy. This entropy plays out as the sun's energy is cycled up from the plants to the herbivores. Due to loss of energy in this process, 1000 units of plants can support only 100 units of herbivores[61]. This also means that the toxins and chemicals found in 1000 units of plants now end up in 100 units of plants. As we move up in the food chain, 100 units of herbivores can support only 10 units of carnivores (humans, sharks, lions, etc.). This means that the toxins and chemicals found in 1000 units of plants are now spread out between 10 humans[62]. Gram for gram, comparing the tissue of humans with plants, you know why herbivores can have more toxins than plants and likewise why humans (or other carnivores) can have more toxins than herbivores. So, if you want to choose an "organic lifestyle," the most efficient and cost-effective way to do this is by choosing to eat mostly plant-based at the lower end of the food chain with the least amount of toxins[63] and chemicals. Fewer toxins entering the body means that the cells generate fewer oxidants (- 'free radicals'). This will limit the number of "bulls" formed in the "China shop" of your cells. A lower amount of cancer-inducing chemicals entering the body (by choosing to eat at the lower end of the food chain) leads to fewer DNA breaks and, hence, less risk for cancer.

R: Let me see if I tracked these details correctly. Cancer is initiated when DNA breaks happen which in turn begin when there is a build up of free radicals in the cell from how the carcinogens interact with the cells. The DNA breaks can be repaired by the cell to an extent. To minimize the load of carcinogens getting into our body, paying attention to the food chain and choosing plant-foods at the lower end of the food chain cuts the load of carcinogens entering our bodies.

B: That sounds right. There is one more thing that is involved with cancer initiation. High protein in the diet creates[64] a temporary build up of a chemical in the cell called epoxide[65] that also contributes to initiating the cancer chain reaction[66].

R: Now I get it about cancer initiation and how we can minimize it from happening in our bodies. How can we figure out what works and what doesn't work to reduce cancer risk? There is so much confusion out there!

B: It is true. Cancer is a complex disease, and the human body, yours truly that is, is too. I am complicated! Once you understand me and my workings better, you will feel empowered to care for your health and prevent cancers. One efficient way to find clues to complex solutions is to find out who are the outliers who are doing better in dealing with a problem and then figure out what is unique about how they deal with it that is making them successful.

R: Reminds me of organizations and how some teams in an organization are successful and others aren't.

B: Exactly. When we study the successful groups, we find out that either they are gifted and have special attributes or they are on the same level playing field but just use different strategies. Let's talk about the risk of cancers in mammals as an example of special attributes. A study in 2015[67] found that elephants have a much lower risk of cancers compared to humans, their fellow mammals. They are so much like humans in many ways. They live in social groups. The groups have a leader. They have immense memory. It is said that elephants, in the wild, can recognize a human years after not seeing each other. Above all, they grieve the loss of a fellow elephant in the group, and they have rituals in the grieving process. But one of the differences between elephants and humans has something to do with cancer risk.

R: How so?

B: Researchers found that humans have only one set of genes called **p53** genes that protect us against cancer. Elephants have twenty sets of these genes[68]. That is what is thought to be the reason why the elephants that were studied showed only a 3% risk of getting cancer. These are captive elephants who live in unnatural settings, are closer to industrialized human communities, and are very likely stressed out. All of these will make them more vulnerable to cancer and even then, they have a very low rate of cancer compared to humans. I would imagine that the cancer risk of elephants in the wild would be even less.

R: That is interesting. So, we have only one set of these p53 genes to protect us? Do they last forever? How can we ensure these genes work at their best to protect us?

B: Researchers studied[69] patients with colon cancer and what breaks their p53 genes regarding their lifestyle behaviors. What showed up was the consumption of total daily meat intake, which includes chicken, turkey, beef, pork, and lamb. For every 5 ounces of these meats consumed daily, the risk of breaking the p53 genes and causing advanced-stage colon cancer went up nearly 3 and a half times! So, it appears that if people reduce consumption of chicken, turkey, beef, pork, mutton, and lamb, colon cancer could be avoided for people who consider what they put in their breakfast, lunch, and dinner for protein.

R: Okay, that sounds like it is a very specific type of cancer you are talking about. Let me play devil's advocate: Has the opposite situation shown to be true. I mean, has eating food with more fruits and vegetables and plant protein shown to improve the p53 gene's work to protect against cancer?

B: I was hoping you would ask. Yes, it has been shown that eating more plant-based foods high in anti-oxidants boost the p53 gene's protection[70].

R: That is interesting to get a clue like that from elephants. I didn't know that animal protein can increase the risk of cancer. Do we have any other such outlier group clues pointing to solutions for how to avoid cancer?

B: Yes. By studying a group of humans who have a genetic syndrome called Laron syndrome. In order to understand how they are immune to cancer, how to minimize the risk in others is best understood by understanding how *step two* of cancer evolves. That step is called "Cancer promotion." It involves meat and dairy as well as excessive levels of estrogen and high levels of something called Insulin-like Growth Factor-1 (IGF-1). I will begin by clarifying what I mean by meat and dairy. Animal protein that comes from chicken, eggs, beef, pork, lamb, fish, cheese, milk, yogurt, and other dairy products promotes cancer. How? They are efficient match-makers who attach the carcinogens to the DNA material of your cells through epoxide bridges. They bring the high-energy bull into the China shop and set them free. They are particularly good at doing that.

Not only does animal protein bring the bull into the China shop, but it also increases the levels of a particular growth promoter to an excessive level, leading to the promotion of cancer. Growth promoter, when in excess, starts promoting tumor growth. We are talking about IGF-1, also called Insulin-like Growth Factor -1. This IGF-1 is essential for growth when you are a kid growing up to be an adult, but once you reach your maximum physical stature in your adulthood, there is no need for increased levels of IGF-1. Rather, such high levels of IGF-1 only increase cancer growth[71, 72].

How do we get increased levels of IGF-1? Researchers have found that intake of animal protein is directly correlated with the amount of IGF-1, with other things remaining constant. The higher the intake of animal protein, the higher the blood level of IGF-1[73]. When looking at risks for getting breast cancer, one of the strongest pieces of evidence confirmed the correlation between the adult-attained height of women and their risk for breast cancer. That is, taller women have a higher risk for breast cancer[74]. Researchers believe that foods chosen during adolescence may have an impact on increasing IGF-1 levels[75, 76] in these women, thereby increasing their risk for breast cancer when they are adults. If this theory is true, then it would mean that not having IGF-1 would make us immune to having cancer, right? What a crazy idea! It may also mean that we would not grow to full adult physical stature in this situation. Is it even possible? Welcome to Laron Syndrome.

R: Never heard of Laron syndrome until this conversation.

B: There is a group of individuals who have a genetic defect that prevents them from having adequate IGF-1 working effectively to grow. So, they remain short-statured without growing to their full potential height. The silver lining in their lives is that these individuals with Laron syndrome are also known to be immune to cancer[77, 78] and diabetes. Both these diseases require IGF-1 to play a role in developing these cancers. So, it is well documented that 1. IGF-1 plays a role in cancer, and 2. diet with animal protein is correlated to higher blood levels of IGF-1. In order to clarify this biological connection between animal protein consumption and cancer, we need to look at populations and their diet and see who is getting high cancer rates or low cancer rates. It is known that Seventh-Day Adventists who abstain from eating animal protein have lower rates of cancer[79, 80, 81] compared with an average population with an average intake of animal protein.

R: So, what do diet and Laron syndrome mean to me? Does this mean if I switch from animal protein to plant protein, a kid will stop growing to her/his full height?

B: A well-planned plant-based diet with a variety of foods that replaces animal protein with plant- protein will provide for normal growth of a kid and, at the same time, reduce her/his risk of getting cancer and diabetes[82]. The problem with folks with Laron syndrome is a genetic defect in the growth factor. A properly balanced plant-based diet can provide an adequate, but not excess, amount of growth factor. This way, growth is not interrupted; only the growth of cancer is not fueled.

R: Okay, I am sold up to this point. But what about breast cancers in women, where their hormones determine the risk of breast cancer? Where does my diet fit into that equation?

B: Great questions. Lack of dietary fiber and excess body weight are the answers. I will explain the role of dietary fiber first. Excessive estrogen activity can increase the growth of certain breast cancers that are sensitive to the effect of excess estrogen. Dietary fiber can keep a check on the estrogen levels from becoming abnormally excessive.

R: How does it do this?

B: I need to first tell you about how estrogen travels in the body in two types. One is attached, and the other is "single." The attached estrogen is bound to a protein called sex hormone binding protein. When estrogen is bound to this protein, it does not stimulate the breast cancer tissue to grow. On the other hand, the "single," unattached estrogen is trouble. It can stimulate the growth of breast cancer cells, especially when in excess[83]. The way the body balances the amount of circulating unattached estrogen molecules is by the amount of sex-hormone binding protein. When more of these proteins are available, they bind to more estrogen, keeping them bound, and thus, there are fewer free, unattached estrogen molecules. This means less trouble with regard to breast cancer. Wouldn't it be nice to have something in our diet that we can consume on a regular basis that can work on this balance system to reduce breast cancer risk? Voila! Dietary fiber. Yes, colorful fruits, vegetables, and beans, naturally rich in dietary fiber, can increase the sex-hormone binding protein[84, 85], thus binding many estrogen molecules. This limits free-floating, unattached estrogen, thus reducing the risk of estrogen-triggered breast cancers. Such a diet rich in plants and dietary fiber also enhances excretion of excess estrogen levels through bile via liver and intestines and out of our system by fecal excretion[86, 87]. It appears that the friendly bacteria in the intestines may have something to do with the effect of fiber on reducing excess estrogen levels[88].

It is also good to remember that alcohol intake can stimulate excess IGF-1 levels in the body.

R: I didn't know that dietary fiber on the meal plate balances hormone levels that impact cancer risk. How does this apply to other cancers like prostate cancer? My uncle died of prostate cancer after going through treatment to keep a check on his testosterone hormone. He hated the treatment because it made him feel less manly in many ways. He developed breasts, became impotent, lost his hair, and got so depressed.

B: Correct. After the diagnosis of prostate cancer, the goal of hormonal therapy is to remove any influence of testosterone on the prostate cancer cells. Suppressing every ounce of testosterone will have the unfortunate side effects he went through. It goes with the territory. That is different from keeping a check on excessive testosterone hormone in the prostate cells by the sex hormone binding protein. Again, the latter is impacted by how much fiber is on the meal plate[89].

R: The colorful fruits and vegetables also came up when discussing anti-oxidants. Things that make the bull snooze in the China shop.

B: It is true that there is more than one reason to indulge in colorful fruits and vegetables. Choosing protein-rich legumes such as beans and lentils also provide anti-oxidants while at the same time replacing the harmful animal protein as in eggs, cheese, milk, coffee creamer, yogurt, chicken, pork, lamb, and beef. Also, colorful fruit and veggies are loaded with "fighto-chemicals," naturally occurring plant-chemicals. They are called "phyto-chemicals," where "phyto" means plants however, I call them "fighto-chemicals" because they are such good fighters against cancers. These naturally occurring plant fighters are different from human-made pesticides, etc.

R: How do these "fighto" things fight cancer?

B: They facilitate the selective death of cancer cells[90, 91]. Now it is time to blow my horn about the amazing technology that I, the human body, possess! The fighto-chemicals work with me to accurately take out the cancer cells and spare the normal cells. I am so proud to say that there is no collateral damage in this fight, contrary to what you may see in certain cancer chemotherapy or radiation treatment or the immense collateral damage that is inevitable in wars with other humans. Bear with me while I touch briefly on the technical aspect of how this works. I have a system that can locate cells that are in their earliest stage of turning into cancer, and I can kill these cells before they multiply into more cancer cells. Sort of nipping it in the cancer bud! The fancy term for this is "apoptosis," also known as "programmed cell death."

R: That sounds far more sophisticated than some cancer drugs, which could cause side effects by affecting adjacent normal cells.

B: The phyto-chemicals do more to protect against cancer. Remember we talked about DNA repair and how each cell in the body has a system to sew up damaged DNA.

R: Yes, I do.

B: The phytochemicals boost the ability of this DNA repair[92] to prevent the DNA glitch from becoming permanent. There is more sophistication to how food can stop cancer from growing and traveling to other parts of the body, what doctors call 'metastasis.' You see, cancer cells are smart in that they figured out how to feed themselves nutrition to keep growing; of course, the excess IGF-1 levels in the blood are boosting this growth as well. The technique cancer cells use is called angiogenesis.

R: Creation of Angio?

B: You got it. Angio means blood vessel. So, angiogenesis means the creation of new blood vessels. Cancer cells do this[93] trick to not only feed themselves with blood and also the nutrition that is packed in the blood, but they also use these blood vessels to travel places.

R: It sounds like they are engineering their own highways to places near and far. That is a kind of genius, working against the body.

B: Tell me about it. There are many sad bodies filled with fear, hopelessness, and a toxic internal environment, unable to do anything about the traveling ability of these cells. No speed bumps or roadblocks in the highways of those unfortunate individuals.

R: How do you beat that kind of sophistication from the cancer cells with food?

B: I tell folks not to underestimate the power and sophistication of food in dealing with cancer and blocking the different steps the cancer cells come up with. Welcome to anti-angiogenesis food.

R: Keep going.

B: Certain foods have been found to have the ability to stop the cancer cells from constructing these new blood vessels[94, 95]. They not only help to starve the cancer cells of blood circulation and nutrition but also cut off their ability to travel to other places. Exciting stuff is coming out of new research on this topic.

Here is the list of anti-angiogenesis foods with some in the list also packing a higher amount of dietary fiber that is good for friendly gut bacteria:

- Blueberries
- Green tea
- Grapes
- Kale
- Berries
- Citrus fruits

- Tomatoes
- Turmeric
- Parsley
- Dark chocolate
- Garlic
- Lavender
- Apples

Make sure you include them in your diet as often as possible! They're delicious as well as cancer-fighting!

R: It is interesting that many in that list also are high in dietary fiber.

B: Correct. That's what I like about plant foods. They nourish and protect me in more than one way. Like minimizing my exposure to excess Methionine in the diet, for instance.

R: What about Methionine? Tell me about it.

B: Methionine is a building block ('amino acid') for protein. It is mainly found in animal foods. Recommended amount of this amino acid in daily diet is around 730 mg for a person who weighs 150 pounds.[96] Research indicates consuming this in excess of the daily need can feed cancer. And most people consume at the cancer risk level. A serving of just four ounce of ground turkey or tuna or steak as part of a meal in a day has more than 1000 mg of Methionine. In the case of pork, it takes 4.2 ounces to deliver 1000 mg. Over the course of the day, depending on other meals and their ingredients, the person is likely to overdose on Methionine, daily, every week and all year.

R: Do we know if cutting back helps?

B: Yes, at least in the cancers such as stomach cancers where this has been studied. It may apply to others cancers as well. Stomach cancer patients cannot eat food, they are given all their nutrition through an intravenous route. This is called Total Parenteral Nutrition. A group of researchers studying advanced stomach cancers did something interesting[97, 98]. Instead of *total* parenteral nutrition, they gave a sub-total nutrition by removing only one nutrient from the mix. And the cancers slowed down. Not only that. The chemotherapy given to these patients was more effective. How is that possible? Why is that when Methionine is removed from the menu, it led to the slowing of the cancer growth?

It is known that when cancer cells are starved of methionine, they cannot grow fast. Understanding this requires that we discuss the basic biology of cell growth and multiplication. Many specialized proteins in our body are responsible for coordinating the behavior and function of how a cell matures and divides into many cells. One of these proteins is called cyclin-dependent kinase[99] proteins, shortly CDK. These CDKs regulate the growth of the cell at more than one point in the process. Limiting the action of CDKs on the cells limits the proliferative growth of these cells – as in cancer[100].

In other instances, it was also noted that limiting Methionine in nutrition led to an increase in the death of cancer cells through a natural process of the body called apoptosis[101,102] The latter is a protective mechanism that the body has to remove harmful cells, such as newly formed cancer cells. Cutting way back on Methionine helps this apoptosis process to kill off cancer cells. Stopping CDK is now a novel strategy to treat cancer. What has this got to do with Methionine and the cancer patients? Limiting Methionine in meals slows cancer by stopping CDK. Other researchers found similar effects in prostate[103,104,105] and pancreatic cancers[106].

Do we eat Methionine? Yes, a lot. The highest concentrations of Methionine are found in fish, poultry, eggs, cheese, beef, pork, and lamb. Among plant foods, some nuts and processed soy protein isolates are high in Methionine.

How do we emulate in our daily meal menu what was tried in the above research using total intravenous nutrition with limits on the amount of Methionine? Can we think of meals without too much Methionine, that is, without as much fish, eggs, poultry, red meat, and dairy as consumed in an average American diet? Meatless Mondays or Methionine-Free Mondays! In that sense, no excess Methionine can mean no metastases!

R: So, how do I go about increasing my fruit, vegetables, and beans while reducing the load of methionine in food? My doctor has told me to eat more vegetables and fruit, but I never managed to follow the recommendation.

B: Most of it is not your fault. Humans are hard-wired to listen to specific instructions and ignore vague ones. The more specific the directions, the more likely a person is likely to follow them[107]. Otherwise, it is too abstract to easily turn it into practical steps to implement successfully in our daily schedule. For beginners, it is a good idea to start filling up at least half your meal plate with at least three colors of vegetables daily.

R: That should be easy.

B: I think so. Pick a color and pick a vegetable. Mix and match so you can get three colors of vegetables in at least half your meals.

R: So, let me summarize so I can make sure I got all of this correct. Colorful fruits, vegetables, and beans protect us from cancer. Animal protein increases our cancer risk. How? Animal protein plays a diabolic matchmaker by bringing the cancer-causing chemicals and our fragile DNA molecules together through epoxide bridges. On the other hand, plant-protein found in beans, lentils, and colorful fruit and vegetables shield us from cancer by at least seven sophisticated mechanisms:

> 1. Snoozing the "bull" in the China shop of our cells with antioxidant rich colorful fruit and vegetables, thus preventing DNA damage.
> 2. Reducing excessive "single" estrogens by increasing the binding protein called sex-hormone binding globulin
> 3. 'Fighto'-chemicals that work with you, the body, to accurately take out early cancer cells and leave the normal cells alone. Zero collateral damage.
> 4. Limit excess animal protein to limit epoxide bridges that damage the DNA.
> 5. Swap animal protein with plant protein like beans and lentils to limit excess IGF-1 so that it won't grow tumors.
> 6. Anti-angiogenic foods stop cancer from feeding itself and traveling. No new blood vessels for cancer cells!
> 7. And, don't feed the cancer with too much methionine.

CHAPTER THREE
UNPOPULAR RESISTANCE: DIABETES

> Seven-word synopsis
> ***Low-fat, fibrous plant foods defuse insulin resistance***

Body: Hola, Alejandro!

Alejandro: Hola! Do I know you?

B: Yes, of course. I am your body. I have been with you for 56 years and 44 days - all your life. We just never talked openly like this before.

A: This is weird. Why am I hearing you? Is my body speaking to me? Am I going crazy?

B: No, you are not crazy. It is the opposite. You did something brilliant, and I came to congratulate you.

A: What are we talking about here?

B: You agreed to sit in this meditation session. And, equally important is that your high blood sugar problems, OUR high blood sugar problems are gone! Due to the shift you made in your diet over the past year, you put a full stop to the high blood sugar levels that had been out of control for 3 years.

A: Really?

B: Yes, your blood sugars are back to under 100. A part of me, and you, called the pancreas is working more effectively because the insulin released by the pancreas is finally operating at its best. The insulin is effective because my 'insulin-resistant' cells are no longer putting up resistance to the insulin's commands to move the sugar from the blood circulation into the cells and organs so that sugar can be used as fuel by these organs.

A: Can you explain the part where the blood sugar gets into the cells?

B: Of course. Blood sugar is the fuel. It needs to get into the cells of tissues and organs to provide energy for activities inside the cells. Similar to how people used to fill up with fuel for their cars in the past, before the arrival of electric vehicles. Those cars are like organ cells. The fuel needs to get into the car for the car to function. Similarly, glucose molecules need to get into the cells to be used as fuel and insulin helps with this[108].

These glucose molecules are derived from the breakdown of the carbohydrates that we eat. Mind you, there are healthy carbohydrates such as vegetables, fruits, legumes, and whole grains, and unhealthy carbohydrates that are from highly processed flour used to make products like white bread, white rice, pastries, etc., as well as sugary drinks and desserts.

A: Can you tell me more about why my organs cannot utilize the sugar molecules floating in my circulation as their fuel? You said something about a resistance?

B: Resistance. Your, I mean our cells and organs went on strike when insulin tried to attach to the cells to open up the doors for the glucose molecules to get into the cells and away from the blood. This strike is called Insulin Resistance[109, 110]. Without open doors, the glucose molecules remain locked out, and more of these molecules pile up outside the locked doors. This is what we call diabetes.

A: That is interesting. What makes the cells go on strike and resist the command of insulin to open the gates to let the blood sugar into the cells?

B: It is driven by two main reasons. One: accumulation of fats inside the muscles and liver[111, 112]. These excess fats mainly come from our food and reach the blood circulation after going through the digestive process. They get into the cells of muscles and liver and trigger an abnormal messaging problem that shuts down the response of cells to open up the gates for blood sugars when insulin is trying to tell the cells to open up.

The second reason at the root of insulin resistance is long-term inflammation from the visceral fat, which spills into the muscles[113]. Without open doors to get in, the glucose molecules are stuck in the circulation and keep piling up with the next meal and the meal after. This naturally increases the blood sugar level. In the meantime, I had to pump more insulin from the pancreas to see if more insulin would make the doors open[114].

A: I wonder if it started all of a sudden.

B: No, it didn't. It happened over several years. I was watching it unfold. I call it the roller-coaster chase. I am so glad because, over the years, my capacity to manage a steady blood glucose level was undermined by what I saw coming into the circulation through the digestive tract. Sugary molecules, fat, and inflammation. I could take that only for so long. I tried my best to stem the problem by putting out more and more insulin. I had to. Even though I know that high insulin levels in the blood (in response to high blood sugar levels) is not healthy for the heart[115, 116, 117]. Even to the degree that it started messing up with your kidney's ability to release excess sodium from the circulation out through the urine, leading to risk of high blood pressure in you[118, 119]. However, I had to go on my routine of squeezing the pancreas to siphon out more insulin when I saw that the sugar level in the blood kept increasing. The sugar level increased because the sugar couldn't get into the cells and organs to be used up as fuel.

A: What is a roller-coaster chase? Sounds like a thriller movie scene.

B: It was a thriller, alright. What I mean by roller-coaster chase is how I have to pump insulin out of your pancreas to chase the blood sugar and bring its level back into normal range. Like an elevator or roller-coaster goes up and down really fast, your blood sugar was hitting highs and lows. One moment it would go up to 380 and then after a couple of hours drop to 100. It is the result of sweet foods that have sugar and processed white starch. I called these 'roller-coaster foods.' In contrast to the healthy whole grains, these processed carbohydrates have dietary fiber removed from them and are physically altered from how they were when on agricultural land. Without fiber, these foods take a joy ride on the roller-coaster[120, 121, 122], up and down. I don't like it. I have to make the pancreas work at break-neck speed to keep up with the highs. In doing so, I have to flood the system by pouring more insulin into the bloodstream, which is a very bad thing for the arteries, including the arteries in the heart. The lining of the arteries is vital to supply life-supporting blood and oxygen to all the organs. These linings (called endothelia) can get messed up by exposure to excessive insulin[123, 124, 125] in the blood stream. So, the bumpy chase by insulin to maintain the balance of fluctuating blood sugar levels is detrimental to the body as a whole, not just for the pancreas and not just for the arteries. Only the taste buds enjoy a fleeting moment of thrill when the sweet, processed food hits the tongue. The brain eats it up and sends pleasure signals to the mind by firing happy signals. Temporarily. Every time your tongue and brain got that sugar fix, I had to work behind the scenes to do damage control. It gets old after a while, you know. Initially, I tried to cope by putting out more insulin by trying to pack away the excess blood glucose into

the liver[126] and away from blood circulation. But I can do only so much for so long. Your food habits remained the same, so the inflammation in our body continued. Additionally, your meals also had high amounts of fat that resulted in excessive fatty acid circulating in the bloodstream. This excess fat got into the liver and muscle cells, triggering the resistance[127] reaction. Inflammation and insulin resistance in the liver and muscles sustained the abnormal insulin-resistant state where the cells went on strike and stopped listening to the insulin's calls to open the cells' doors to let the glucose in. In the meanwhile, I got exhausted from trying to deploy various coping tactics to keep you in a normal health status. After a point, I just couldn't keep up with the constant need for fixing the problem. I went from being balanced to a state of imbalance. That is when you got diabetes, and your blood sugars started going through the roof.

A: I remember that. My doctor was concerned when he first told me that I had diabetes.

B: Yes, I remember it too. The sugar level was 417. I knew that would also affect other parts of the body.

A: Which parts?

B: Heart, kidneys, eyes, nerves, and a whole bunch of other organs. I was worried for many parts of me and you as we were floating in that sea of blood sugar of more than 400. Our body was crumbling in slow motion. I couldn't help much because every day, my efforts to correct the problem were defeated regularly – during breakfast, lunch, and dinner and whenever you would snack. We were not too far from developing new blood vessels in the retina in the eye.

A: Would it be bad for that to happen?

B: Yes, not good at all. The retina helps you see things. Anything involving new growth, including that of new blood vessels, is going to get in the way of how the visual sensors can work to pick up images that we see and get that information to your brain so that we know what we are seeing. So, when new blood vessels start to grow in the retina, patients get a retinal disease called retinopathy, which correlates with how uncontrolled the blood sugar level is. That is why doctors recommend diabetic patients to get an annual eye check-up to catch this early. Not only the eyes but your heart was at risk as well. The risk for heart attack is much higher among the diabetic population compared to groups with normal blood sugar. The blockage of arteries leading to heart attacks is more pronounced and rapid in diabetics[128].

A: I didn't realize that I was in such big trouble. What was wrong with my kidneys?

B: Well, a few more years and your kidneys would have failed. You were showing early warning signs because your kidneys were beginning to fail in filtering the protein properly. Normally, with someone whose kidneys are working perfectly fine, the kidneys would be able to hold most of the protein back to the blood and not let much of the protein escape the filter and get into the urine. In other words, the amount of protein (albumin) in the urine is usually minimal when the kidneys work well. In your case, the diabetes was messing with the beautiful and strong architecture of the kidneys' filtration system, and so the kidneys were beginning to spill more albumin into the urine. That is an early sign of the troublesome hands of diabetes touching the kidneys. If that had continued for a few more years, the kidneys would have started to shut down, and the individual can live only by a lifeline hooked up to their body three times a week, known as dialysis. Not an ideal quality of life. Additionally, to keep the person alive with the weekly dialysis schedule, there are many resources (mechanical and human) put into that very high-cost effort. Whoever is picking up the tab for the dialysis is in for a sticker shock.

A: I am so glad I changed my eating habits and avoided getting into that mess!

B: You not only escaped that mess but also avoided getting your nerves into trouble[129]. The nerves in the arms, hands, legs, and feet are tiny, and they depend on blood vessels called arteries to deliver oxygen and nutrition. When blood sugar remains high, even just over 100, for many months, it starts to mess with blood circulation for these nerves. You feel it when you feel numbness, tingling, or "pins and needles," like feeling in hands, arms, legs, or feet. Not only that, but diabetes can also affect a whole other system of nerves called autonomic nerves that affect your digestive system and shut off warning signal systems in the body.

A: I have heard John at the office complain that he gets numbness, and his doctor told him that he has "neuropathy." I better tell him to get his blood sugar checked. What is this autonomic nervous system? What happens to the warning signal system in the body?

B: You can call it the automatic nervous system. I totally depend on it for a lot of my automatic functions where I don't have to think, plan, and act. When you feel afraid, I get your heart rate up immediately because of these autonomic nerves. I can have you salivate the moment you witness a delicious meal or even think of it. I can get you to sweat when fearful or have your mouth get dry in a few seconds when you are standing in front of a crowd to speak. I can get your stomach and intestines to contract and move periodically to propel food forward and assist with digestion. I can even get your pupils to open widely when you see your loved one or friend after a long time to take in as much visually as possible. That's my, I mean our, autonomic nervous system. I don't like how high blood sugar messes with my performance. When blood sugar is high, my automatic nervous system, YOUR automatic nervous system, gets all messed up[130]. I can't even send pain signals to warn a person when they are getting a heart attack. Heard of a silent heart attack[131]?

A: Yes, I have. That is scary that one can't even feel the pain of a heart attack.

B: The good news is that you avoided a whole lot of these troubles by switching your diet and reversing diabetes. I am happy I am dealing with blood sugars around 90-100 in your case these days. You did it!

A: Initially, it was hard for me to think of another way of doing things. I was feeling tired and didn't have the energy to do all that I wanted to do, so I was barely making it through the daily stuff I had to finish to keep my job going. I had house construction commitments with my clients that I had to finish to get their checks to pay my bills. I was eating what I was used to: chicken, beef roast, fish, white rice, and soda. Lots of milk, too. It was interesting that I had the feeling to decline medications or insulin for diabetes when I was diagnosed with it.

B: As I always say, ideally insulin ought to come from within, through the body's natural mechanisms - my system - not from a pharmacy.

A: When I declined medications and insulin, my doctor said that there was hope. He initially asked me to increase my vegetable intake – both the portions and the types of vegetables I was eating. He said it doesn't matter whether they are cooked or they are raw but asked me to eat at least half of the veggies as raw salads. He asked me to cut out red meat (beef, pork, lamb), dairy and eggs.

B: Was it hard to do?

A: It was for the first week, then I got used to it. I was also determined to take care of myself without depending on drug companies. In two weeks, my blood sugar dropped to 300.

B: Yes, I was able to do a better job in trying to fire up the exhausted pancreas to work better with your own insulin. And the cells and organs were also beginning to get (literally) attached to the insulin. The 'open sesame' command by those insulin molecules worked better because the cells were starting to listen to the insulin to open the doors for glucose molecules to enter the cells and leave the blood circulation. That way, the cells can start to use the glucose molecules as fuel for energy.

A: It makes sense. I could feel my energy level returning within a few weeks of changing my meals.

B: Correct. Your energy level bounced back because the cells could finally make use of the glucose fuel.

A: Cutting out the chicken and cheese was the hardest because I was eating plenty of them.

B: I remember those days. Your meals were heavy with poultry, and cheese kept the inflammation machinery in full swing. And the eggs you ate for breakfast every day certainly didn't help[132].

A: I don't know. I was told by my buddy to eat more protein and limit carbohydrates. He had diabetes, and he told me to eat eggs to avoid diabetes.

B: How did you manage to omit the chicken, eggs, and cheese, then? Some people find it hard to give up the habit of eating them, especially cheese.

A: I started to use more beans in my dishes. Rice with beans and veggies. I flavored it with some taco flavoring. Even in salads, I would throw in a cup of chickpeas or white beans. Quitting cheese was a pain in the neck. I got very anxious about quitting cheese, almost like an addict trying to quit his addiction. What made me quit was the fact I truly recognized the scale of how much cheese was part of my meals and my life. It was in everything, and I never noticed that it was virtually in all my food. Cheese was part of tacos, burgers, burritos, lasagna, pasta, sandwiches, snacks, and so on. I actually started writing down the list of foods that had cheese in them, and that did it for me. The list became endless, and it just spooked me that I didn't realize how big a part cheese was playing in my life. It was almost like the cheese was controlling my meal routine rather than the other way around. That realization made me reconsider my choices. The cheese went out the window, and so did the chicken and their eggs. I started eating more veggies and beans. Switched up the rice to brown rice and reduced the portion size while replacing snacks with fruit. No more soda and candies. My blood sugar dropped to 100 in a few months, and I kept it that way. It has been over a decade, since I got the sugar down to 100.

B: Do you miss the cheese?

A: I did miss cheese initially, but now I am over it. However, I am becoming fond of this recipe from a lady who hired me for a house extension job. She told me about making a delicious cheese sauce without the cheese.

B: Glad you found that one.

A: From what I heard from you, it looks like it is not all about carbohydrates. Not only that, it seems like carbohydrates in their whole form and not processed could be helpful after all because of the dietary fiber they bring along with them onto the meal plate.

B: Correct. Of course, highly processed carbohydrates and sugary foods are a problem. There are some other equally if not more problematic areas in the food landscape that haven't gotten as much scrutiny and censure as sugary snacks have. For instance, excess dietary fats, both of animal and plant origin, can get into the liver and muscles and activate insulin resistance. Protein from an animal source lacks the key ingredient, dietary fiber, that could help keep the gut lining from firing up long-term inflammation, which could worsen insulin resistance[133]. Compare protein from plants such as legumes, whole grains, nuts, seeds, and, yes, vegetables - all bring along a good dose of dietary fiber, as long as they are not processed.

A: I didn't realize that dietary fiber is a special part of a healthy meal.

B: Dietary fiber plays a central role in maintaining normal glucose levels and ideal body weight through multiple tactics.

First off, dietary fiber in the meals makes sure that there is a steady supply of hormone produced in the intestines called Glucagon-like Peptide-1 (GLP-1). This hormone is vital to maintain appetite control and reduce food cravings. GLP-1 is also helpful in maintaining the optimal amount of insulin release from the pancreas to maintain normal blood glucose levels. Dietary fiber stimulates the intestinal cells to produce sufficient quantities of GLP-1[134, 135]. Besides helping with its production, dietary fiber also helps limit the destruction of GLP-1 in the body. There are certain enzymes in the body that naturally break down the GLP-1 and remove them from the body. These enzymes are called Dipeptidyl peptidase-4 (DDP-4) enzymes. If something can deter this enzyme from breaking down the GLP-1, that will help maintain a steady availability of this hormone to maintain blood sugar and curb excess appetite. Well, the dietary fiber in unprocessed plant foods can do just that. They stop this DDP-4 enzyme. You might have heard of pharmaceutical medications that have taken a leaf out of the fiber book to create prescription medications that mimic GLP-1 or stop the DDP-4 enzyme, all aimed at regulating blood sugar levels to normal levels. Dietary fiber has been doing these tasks for ages, in a natural way, before these drugs were discovered. Additionally, some of the antioxidants in some of these plant foods also exert the same beneficial effect through different mechanisms[136].

The second tactic that dietary fiber uses to maintain normal blood sugar is ingenious. It has to do with a concept called gluconeogenesis[137], which simply means creating glucose molecules from non-starch raw material such as protein. Yes, I can make new glucose molecules without carbohydrates or starch as a raw material. For instance, I can use amino acids, the building block of protein, to create new glucose molecules. This process resulting in *glucose-newly-created* in this way is called *gluco-neo-genesis*. Get it?

A: I am following the logic in the name. But I am not following the logic of how making more new glucose will help with controlling diabetes. It sounds counter-intuitive, don't you think?

B: You are correct, but I haven't told you the full story yet! Now, when such gluconeogenesis happens in the intestinal cells, it sends up a signal through the blood channels to the brain's appetite regulation headquarters. This results in the person feeling satisfied with the meal and no longer hungry. Dietary fiber, found in leafy greens, vegetables, fruit, legumes, and whole grains, stimulates the production of intestinal gluconeogenesis, resulting in appetite control from the brain. Of note, when people are doing intermittent fasting, the intestines kick into gluconeogenesis[138], which results in better control over cravings.

The third tactic deployed by the dietary fiber is through a special set of fatty acids called Short Chain Fatty Acids (SCFAs). These are produced when the dietary fiber is fermented by the healthy gut bacteria[139]. Most of the SCFAs are produced in the upper section of the colon near the junction where the small intestine meets the colon. A small percentage of these SCFAs are reabsorbed back into the bloodstream to produce an array of benefits for the body's health, including anti-inflammatory, anti-cancer, anti-microbial, and stability of the gut's defense barrier. One of the metabolic functions that is achieved after a few months by these SCFAs is the regulation of blood sugar control[140]. Without enough dietary fiber in the meals, it is hard to produce these beneficial SCFAs to make a beneficial impact on blood glucose.

A: /*Guau.*

B: There's more. Bile acid flows through the liver, gets concentrated in the gall bladder, and then gets introduced into the intestines, where most of them are reabsorbed back into the same flow cycle. These bile acids and gut microbiomes are mutually linked and affect each other. Dietary fiber in the meals ensures that the healthy bacteria thrive and produce a second variety of bile acids called secondary bile acids. These activate a specific type of docking station in the cell's nucleus called [141] Farnesoid X Receptors (FXR). Such activation has been implicated in beneficial effects on diabetes, inflammatory bowel disease, and colorectal cancer protection.

Something notable is that of all the plant foods, leafy greens have been shown to be the most powerful in working against diabetes. For every additional serving of leafy greens, your risk of diabetes drops by 14%[142] (one serving of spinach = 2 cups of uncooked spinach). Leafy greens are not only a source of dietary fiber, vitamins, minerals, antioxidants and phytochemicals but also contain omega-3 fatty acids, a type of anti-inflammatory compound. Alpha-linolenic acid, a type of omega-3 fatty acid found in leafy greens, strengthens the walls of the cells that control the movement of blood glucose molecules. Omega-3 fatty acids also have an anti-inflammatory effect to reduce insulin resistance[143].

A: I had no idea that dietary fiber is so vital for controlling diabetes. I have also heard about carbohydrate count and that one is supposed to track carbohydrate count.

B: Counting dietary fiber count is equally, if not more important than counting carbohydrate count. The carbohydrate count that comes in a wholesome package along with dietary fiber is less ominous than the carbohydrate count from sugary or processed carbohydrate food sources that are devoid of dietary fiber.

A: When I wasn't eating well, I felt like an old man. I had no energy. I was slow and pretty much degenerating. Was that related to the inflammation?

B: Partly due to the long-term inflammation. It was also due to A.G.E.

A: Do you mean my age?

B: I meant A.G.E., an acronym for Advanced Glycated End-products. They are proteins that have a structural change due to a 'glycosyl' molecule attached to them, which comes from age and high sugar in the cell's surrounding environment. The latter happens when there are excess blood sugar levels. What is striking is that when the body has more of these proteins attached to the 'glycosyl' molecules, that person's body starts to age faster. Coincidentally, A.G.E. is associated with aging faster[144]. One way to think about it is to see diabetes as an aging disease[145]. When diabetes is out of control, that person is aging faster.

Another way A.G.E. increases in our body and increases our age is through foods, especially related to cooking them at very high temperatures to the extent that they are charred or burned; Especially with animal foods.[146,147]

A: Interesting. I have never heard of these Advanced Glycated Proteins.

B: You have heard of something very similar in its nature, but just not with that exact name. Has your doctor ever asked you to check your diabetes control by checking the blood levels of 'Hemoglobin A1C'?

A: Yes, twice a year.

B: Well, the other name for that test is 'Glycosylated Hemoglobin.' Here hemoglobin is the protein that gets the glycosyl molecule attached to it. Hemoglobin is the red pigment protein that gives the color for the red blood cells that carry oxygen in the blood circulation. This 'glycosylated hemoglobin' aka 'Hemoglobin A1C' test is not only an indicator of blood sugar control but also about how fast the body is aging[148,149].

A: Well, when my doctor started treating my diabetes, my A1C test was 12%, and I was told that the normal is under 6.5%. I was 40 years old then. Does that mean I was aging then?

B: Correct, the calendar would have shown that you were 40 years old then, but inside, your tissues and organs were beginning to behave more like a 50-year-old's, or an even older person. Luckily, you put an end to that fast-track aging process by cleaning up your diet to improve your diabetes and A1C numbers. Not only that, but you also reduced your risk of dementia and memory loss setting in down the line[150, 151, 152, 153, 154].

A: I didn't know diabetes was connected to dementia. I guess I didn't even know the things that I was protecting myself from by eating more wholesome, fiber-rich vegetables and legumes.

B: The connection between uncontrolled diabetes in the middle years and dementia later in life is strongly established through science. So much so that some in the medical research world call Alzheimer's dementia as Type 3 Diabetes[155, 156, 157, 158, 159].

A: Type 3 Diabetes? Never heard of such a thing! Tell me more about this connection with diabetes.

B: Let's touch on some basics about the brain and blood sugar. Brain cells need fuel to function. The only fuel they can use is carbohydrates. Brain cells cannot make use of protein or fats because these two entities don't have the password to enter the brain cells. Only carbohydrates have the ability to cross the barrier between the brain cells and the blood circulation[160] so that glucose molecules can enter the brain cells to be used as fuel. Imagine how much starvation one's brain goes through if someone is on a no-carbohydrate or low-carbohydrate diet! Many get on the latest diet hype that cuts out most or all carbohydrates, even the wholesome dietary fiber and anti-oxidant-rich carbohydrates. That is not at all healthy for the brain. It will cause clouded, foggy thinking in the short term and memory loss in the long run. Choosing healthy, wholesome carbohydrate sources not only helps fight diabetes through fiber content but also feeds the brain cells properly and avoids the risk of memory loss. It is very clear that brain cells are sensitive to changes in the amount of glucose molecules in the cell's neighborhood. Both high and low blood sugars are detrimental to the brain cells[161]. Uncontrolled blood sugar, in the long run, has been shown to create an imbalance in insulin levels. Such insulin imbalance is a hallmark of changes in the brain cells in Alzheimer's dementia. The molecular findings in the cells are identical with regard to diabetes and Alzheimer's disease. Insulin imbalance is key for the formation of 'amyloid plaques,' the hallmark changes noticed in the brain of Alzheimer's patients, as well as the characteristic 'neurofibrillary tangles' in the brain of such patients. The amyloid, a.k.a. senile plaques, are found outside the nerve cells of the brain. The tangles are abnormal clumps of filament-shaped Tau proteins that are normally found inside the nerve cells as part of the cell's structural framework. The insulin imbalance signature is found all over the place in the tangles and the senile plaques - the two typical changes that happen as part of the development of Alzheimer's dementia.

A: Let me see if I can summarize. In essence, insulin resistance in the liver and muscles can lead to Type 2 diabetes, and insulin resistance in the brain can lead to Alzheimer's dementia. Hence, the name Type 3 Diabetes for such dementia. Sweet new memories may not be stored in the brain due to sweets. Even pre-diabetes associated with long-term inflammation during middle age has been shown to increase the risk of dementia after 20 years.

B: Correct.

A: That's disconcerting to think that I would have been on the path to dementia if I had continued on the original eating habits of soda, sugars, high fat, high animal protein, low fiber diet.

B: You were in the right place at the right time to hear this information from your doctor that got you to switch up to eating more vegetables, beans, and leafy greens and move away from sugars, soda, and animal foods.[162, 163, 164, 165, 166, 167, 168, 169, 170, 171]

A: I am happy that my doctor talked about eating beans and veggies. I wish my friend's doctor had introduced this idea of eating whole, plant-based food to prevent his diabetes. He knows that I controlled my blood sugars to under 100, and yet he argues with me about the food. His doctor is also not talking about it. You would think that doctors would want to talk about this.

B: Well, doctors are a group of caring professionals who have compassion and good intentions and work with the training and tools they have. Their toolbox handed to them from their training period lacks the nutrition tool. They have got some pretty nifty tools and a matching competence to save someone from trauma, medical and emergencies like when something breaks in the body. When I am the body of someone who got into a vehicle crash or fell off a ladder, I am so happy that the medical doctors can save me and my body parts. Interestingly enough, the same level of finesse and high-tech mechanisms are present in how healthful food heals our bodies from long-term diseases. Students in medical schools barely receive any nutrition training so we understand their lack of knowledge.

A: I hope the medical school training starts to include more nutrition classes.

B: Do you know how many hours of nutrition education are required of medical schools in the US? Approximately 24 hours. In all their 4 years of medical school. So, doctors, when they graduate from medical schools, are short-changed by not having been given the adequate knowledge to handle diseases of nutrition. Most of the chronic diseases that make up a big part of healthcare's burden are related to diet. In fact, an analysis looked at 17 leading risk factors that contribute to death and disabilities among Americans and listed them according to the scale of the effect[172].

Guess which one took the number one title for causing the most deaths and disabilities among Americans? Dietary factors! Not drugs, not lack of physical activity, not even tobacco. Despite the fact that diet and nutrition play such a fundamental role in a large set of diseases that account for more than 85% of today's healthcare expenditure, there is barely any nutrition education for students of today's medical schools.

A: Talking about expenditure, my buddy spends nearly $220 every month on medical supplies for testing blood sugar and for his insulin and pills to control his blood sugar. That's $2,640 per year. If one takes all the diabetics in this country, then you would see some are spending more and some less based on how bad their blood sugar is. I read in an email that the American Diabetic Association claims that when we take all the diabetics in this country and average their out-of-pocket expenditure, it comes to more than $12,000 per capita annually. If you think about it, I dodged spending $2,640 yearly for the past 10 years. That would be $26,400. That is a lot of money I would rather spend on renovating my house, paying off my debts, or taking a few vacations - all made possible by going to whole, plant-based food like my doctor advised me to.

B: That is quite a big chunk of money you saved by eating well. That is a nice return for choosing to eat well.

A: Not only that. The bigger deal for me is that I have control over my body's health. My health is in my hands. Do you know how powerful that feeling is? Well, you do because we are the same.

B: Why does that matter to you that much?

A: I have my independence in this lifestyle of eating healthy. I don't stand in line in the pharmacy. I don't worry about co-pays for my medications or insulin. It is like driving your own car. I am in the driver's seat.

B: What is the role of the doctor when someone has diabetes or a similar long-term medical condition, in your opinion?

A: In my ideal world, they are coaches and guiding partners in my journey toward health. They would provide the latest and most accurate information regarding how to take care of one's own health using nutrition, physical activity, and stress management, motivate me when I am slipping. Equally important is that they make me realize my full potential by taking my health into my own hands. In my situation, I feel I have the knowledge and self-management skills to take care of my diabetes by way of my lifestyle. And that is such an empowering gift. Before we wrap up here, let me summarize what we discussed:

1. Insulin resistance is caused by fat buildup in liver and muscles and from excess inflammation – all related to excess dietary fats.
2. Processed carbohydrates/sugars, high fats, and protein without dietary fiber – all contribute to diabetes.
3. Dietary fiber (greens, vegetables and beans) regulates appetite, increases meal satisfaction, and limits over consumption by feeding the microbiome which releases GLP-1 to regulate appetite, body weight, and blood sugar.
4. Dietary fiber and gut bacteria control blood pressure through kidney's ability to reabsorb sodium.
5. For every additional leafy green serving, diabetes risk drops by 14%.
6. Multiple organs are impacted by uncontrolled diabetes.
7. Type 3 diabetes – Alzheimer's disease and diabetes link.
8. A.G.E. and hemoglobin A1C – both are markers of aging.

CHAPTER FOUR
UNTANGLING THE GORDIAN KNOT: HEART HEALTH

> Seven-word synopsis
> *Oil-free, wholefood plant meals open blocked arteries*

Jason: Why did this happen to me at this time in my life?

B: What are you talking about?

J: My heart attack that happened a month ago. I have too much happening in my life currently, and I don't have time for a heart attack. It is tax return season, and many of my usual clients are still collecting the necessary paperwork to file the tax return request.

B: Correct. Many people don't have time for unwinding these days. Keep going with what you were saying.

J: At age 47, I am looking at the possibility of my teenage kids going to college in a few years. And my niece is graduating post-graduate college soon. I have been at my current job as accountant for fifteen years, and my career is going well. In fact, the prospects of getting a promotion are looking good in the near future. My wife and I have no time for ourselves because we both are putting in sixty-plus hours per week to pay the mortgage, put the kids through school, and save money for college. And now this. Having a heart attack is affecting my schedule. I was fortunate last month that I had a stent put in as a rescue measure. Still, I am worried about my plans for the future.

B: I can see how this can be so upsetting. I feel the same pain you do. After all, I am you, and you are me.

J: I know. The pain I felt during the heart attack was extraordinary, something that I have never felt before. It was like someone was, something was….

B: ………sitting on your chest? I know. That was a first experience for me in our journey together. I had difficulty pushing the blood to where your heart needed oxygen badly. I tried my best, but it was impossible with the blockage in the artery. Up until that unfortunate day, the heart artery was developing the blockage slowly over decades and got to a stage of partially blocking the plumbing. I was trying to prevent that catastrophe by keeping a protective lid ('fibrin cap[173]') over the partial blockage, thus insulating it from the blood cells in the river of blood flowing right next to it. I knew that if that cap broke open, then all hell would break loose, resulting in an instant heart attack. All my efforts to keep the protective cap were being challenged by the inflammation[174] building up in the neighborhood and all over your body. I wish you knew that all your over-indulgence in your breakfast, lunch, and dinner were not helping me keep the lid on the impending crisis. Additionally, I was also trying to build new detour roads ('anastomosis) in the form of parallel plumbing channels in case the blockage became total so that at least some of the traffic, i.e., oxygen/blood flow, could keep flowing through the detour channels.

J: I had no idea of all the things you were doing to protect me. I feel very grateful. I want to learn more and reciprocate with changes that will take care of you.

B: On that day, the protective cap gave out due to unrelenting inflammation, exposing the blood cells to the core of the partial blockage. That is all it took for the blockage to become one hundred percent, total clogging of the artery in a matter of minutes, shutting off all blood flow and its oxygen load to downstream heart muscles. I tried my best, but it felt like I was pushing against a wall in vain. How can I supply the oxygen to the heart muscle where it is most needed when I can't get the blood cells to flow past the hundred percent? And, my backup crew that usually steps in during such times, was down as well.

J: What backup crew? Also, we need to discuss the food indulgences you said were not helping you.

B: Yes, I will get to the food in detail soon. First, about the backup crew. They are my cells that coat the lining of the plumbing ('artery') through which the oxygen-rich blood is flowing like a river. Scientists and medical professionals call them 'endothelial cells'[175] - they usually come to the rescue whenever there is a need to push a higher volume of blood through the blood circulation. On-demand, they basically open the girth of the arterial plumbing, making it wide enough to allow for additional blood flow. This rescue crew was weak, in your case, made lame by the type of food you were eating[176]. It didn't have to be that way if you had been made aware of the importance of paying more attention to your lifestyle to prevent the heart attack in the first place[177,178,179,180,181,182,183,184,185] or its complications such as heart failure[186].

J: What went wrong? I thought I was healthy and doing all the right things. I switched most of my red meat intake to chicken, had healthy eggs for breakfast, and stopped smoking cigarettes.

B: I am so grateful you stopped those nasty cigarettes. They were choking me, and I couldn't stand how people would smell the cigarettes on you and try to avoid you all the while when you had no clue as to how you smelled of nicotine. The success you had with changing your cigarette habits is the same kind of success you would want for your food.

J: What am I doing wrong with my food? I have been eating this same way for ten or eleven years, so why, all of a sudden, did I have a heart attack now?

B: Yes, you tried for eleven years after tinkering with the diet from how it used to be when you were growing up. That tinkering around the edges wasn't enough. You weren't sufficiently educated about what else you needed to change. While you were pruning your diet at the edges, I felt the inflammation march on unchecked.

J: What inflammation? Where?

B: All over you - and me, of course. When talking about how inflammation and heart attacks occur, it is specifically in the arteries in your heart where the warning sign happens before the heart attack itself. Remember, you were holding your chest and had that suffocating feeling of not being able to breathe? That was the tip of the iceberg. The iceberg was building over years, even decades.

J: I remember that horrible feeling of tightness in my chest. I felt helpless.

B: I have all the tools in place to make sure you don't get into that kind of situation again, however, the diet you were eating was just too much for me to cope with, so I finally gave in. And we had that heart attack.

J: What tools? How is that connected to my diet?

B: I am talking about the trinity of the endothelium, nitric oxide, and anti-oxidants.

J: Heard of anti-oxidants but not nitric oxide? Isn't that nitric oxide that makes you laugh?

B: No, that is nitrous oxide – laughing gas. This one is nitric oxide, no laughing matter. I love this one. It makes arteries open up when needed so I can pump more blood to any organ when I need.

J: I think you said that the endothelium was a series of cells coating the inner lining of the plumbing that carries healthy, oxygen-rich blood.

B: Correct. The arteries. When the inner coating cells are healthy without cholesterol or inflammation coming from unhealthy food and smoking, these endothelial cells pump out nitric oxide on demand to keep the oxygen flowing in the blood to wherever it is needed. When unhealthy foods[187, 188] and/or nicotine[189] hurt this inner coating, nitric oxide is not pumped out, and there is no adequate blood flow when the demand increases in a particular area of the organ, such as the heart muscle or, for that matter, any organ where good flow of blood matters.

J: If it is the same phenomenon in other organs, is that why I had erectile issues for the past few years?

B: Yes, but not only the blood flow to your genital organs. The same thing applies to blood flow to the heart, brain, and other vital organs. See, the arteries in you form a total system, as in a tree. So, if there is nourishment and vitality in the tree, then it will show up in all the branches, whether the branch is in the leg or heart or wherever. Likewise, if the tree is diseased, all branches dwindle and fail to work. That is why erectile dysfunction is a precursor of heart attacks[190, 191] waiting to happen. With diseases in arteries across the body, when your heart needs more blood flow when you are walking or doing something strenuous, the diseased artery cannot produce enough nitric oxide to open up the artery more to allow for additional blood to run through it. This leads to a supply and demand problem. There is a demand for more blood flow, but the supply is not reaching the target location because the pipeline (artery) cannot be made wider to supply more blood. The lack of oxygen in such a crisis is felt as pain. That is what you felt that day in your chest. When the endothelial cells don't make nitric oxide, it is like working with a straight jacket to open up a closed oxygen tank when the oxygen is a dire need.

J: Not sure if I am following all of what you just said. Can you come at it from another angle and elaborate a bit more about how this endothelium has something to do with the nitric oxide? Where do blocked arteries fit into this picture?

B: Well, both the issues of failed endothelial production of nitric oxide and blocked arteries are connected. The endothelial cells form the lining of the interior surface of the arteries that come in contact with the blood. Imagine a plumbing system. The inner surface of the pipeline comes in contact with the water in the plumbing. Similarly, the inner lining of the arteries comes in contact with blood. Now imagine that the arteries are just branches of an entire tree of circulation. All the inner linings, if healthy, can open up the plumbing by widening the tubes when there is a need for more blood flow. The inner lining of arteries gets diseased with a poor diet. This leads to an abnormal collection of cholesterol at one spot in the artery[192, 193].

J: How does this begin? What happens early on in that bad spot where the artery gets blocked?

B: I try my best to keep the arteries clean and running well. However, due to what we eat, I end up with inflammation all over the body, and in my teenage years, my body developed a small weak point in one of the arteries in the heart. This weak point attracts white blood cells to the area to try and clean up the mess. Not only that. It starts to pull cholesterol molecules like a magnet, especially when there is more cholesterol floating in the blood circulation rather than staying outside the circulation.

J: What do you mean by outside the circulation?

B: The issue with cholesterol is its location. Cholesterol by itself isn't a bad thing.

J: I have always been told to watch out for cholesterol! This is confusing.

B: Yes, but there are some nuances to it. "Watch out for *excess* cholesterol in blood circulation" is a more accurate warning. Here's why! We do need cholesterol because it serves as a raw material to make a lot of our body's steroid hormones[194, 195]. Without cholesterol, my hormonal system would stop working, and I would die! That means you and anyone I am "embodying" will, too.

J: That is news to me!

B: So, it isn't that all cholesterol is bad. The problem is in transportation and storage beyond capacity. First, let's look at the transportation problem. I have some special couriers called 'ABC transporter proteins'[196, 197].

J: What do you mean, ABC proteins? Are you just making up names as you go along?

B: I know the name sounds like I made it up. Really, they are called ABC transporter proteins, and they work like couriers to transport cholesterol molecules[198, 199] in the proper route. The route is always one way - out of the circulation and into either the intestines[200] or the liver.[201] When there is excess cholesterol, the excess gets pushed out into the intestinal system, where it is excreted in the stool. Some of it gets stored in the liver, where it is used as a raw material to make steroid hormones. When there is excess inflammation[202, 203,204] in the body, these ABC proteins stop doing their courier job of eliminating excess cholesterol via our intestine, which leads to fat accumulation in the liver. When the issue continues, the cholesterol starts to build in the circulation because there is only so much that can be stashed away in the closet called 'liver.' It is like how if you have so much junk stuff in the house with a guest is arriving, there is only so much closet space (liver) in which you can stash them away and the rest is going to be in the living room showing up where you don't want them to be (circulation/arteries). An example of how food choices drive inflammation higher is the balance of omega-3 fats and omega-6 fats in the meals[205]. Omega-3 is a powerful ally and is packaged with healthy dietary fiber in the form of flax seeds[206], walnuts, and leafy greens. Omega-6 fats are found in cooking oils and are not so healthy when consumed in excess of omega-3 fats. Consuming more flax and greens and cutting out or cutting way back on the oil helps balance the healthy ratio between omega-3 and omega-6 fats. Without this balance, inflammation fires up on all cylinders. Which means the cholesterol level in the blood builds up. This excess cholesterol floating in the blood gets stuck to the weak point in the artery lining and starts to build up as a blockage. It is the gunk that I don't like. It's gross and awful. I wish the people whom I live in would wake up to this reality and start cleaning up their arteries by eating more such anti-inflammatory meals.

J: So, let me see if I can get this straight. The fact that I ate processed food and animal protein led to increased inflammation in the body. This messed up the ABC couriers badly enough to stop them from doing their job, resulting in more cholesterol getting built up in my circulation. Some of the cholesterol molecules got stuck to the weak point in the artery and started to build up gunk. You tried to put a cap on the developing clog to prevent a catastrophe. My meals were fueling the inflammation[207] issues to the point where your protective lid was ripped off, leading to rapid total clogging of the plumbing. This instantly cut off my heart's oxygen, and I was gasping for oxygen when you were trying to help me with a weakened rescue crew called endothelium that couldn't open the oxygen flow. I ended up with a heart attack then. Am I right?

B: Precisely. You summarized the events well. We covered almost all of the players in this scene.

J: Why 'almost'? Are there more players?

B: Well, there are some good folks we haven't talked about who come to the rescue. Anti-oxidants! Yes, the same ones we hear about when people talk food and reducing the risk of cancer.

J: They seem to help us in many ways. Where can I get them again?

B: Colorful fruit and vegetables. Also, some legumes such as lentils, beans; spices such as cloves & turmeric, and plain cacao without the milk and sugar. Yes, these anti-oxidants help[208] with the oxidative stress that happens in the weak point of the artery's lining. When there are more colorful fruits and vegetables in my people's bodies, I am happy because I can tend to the injuries that happen in these arteries using the anti-oxidants from these wonderful fruits and vegetables. In fact, research has shown that heart disease with blockage in arteries is a disease of deficiency. A deficiency of anti-oxidants in our meals[209]. So, in a way we have a diet of deprivation where we include limited choices of anti-oxidant food in our meals. It hurts, literally. And it's that simple (to fix).

J: Did you say that these events had been going on for decades?

B: Yes. Let's say that I am the living, breathing body of a healthy child. All my organs are in top shape. As the child grows, I get exposed to food that the child likes, but I don't. These are animals turned into food such as fish sticks, chicken, yogurt, cow's milk, eggs, or just sugars and oil and grains stripped off fiber to leave processed grains or just sugar. Collectively, these foods work together over the years to damage the endothelial cell's ability to make nitric oxide when the kid grows to be an adult[210] and needs that nitric oxide to open up the circulation when their heart needs more blood and oxygen.

J: Wow, looks like there are many players in this game!

B: Yes, and I haven't even told you about the other billions of players.

J: Billions? Who?

B: The billions of bacteria in our intestines.

J: What have they got to do with heart arteries? Isn't the gut system separate from the heart system?

B: Remember, everything in me is directly or indirectly connected to one another. I want to introduce you to TMAO – it is a technical word that is a mouthful. Trimethylamine-N-oxide[211]. To keep it simple, we will just refer to it as TMAO. Now, this substance messes with the arteries in the heart and clogs up the artery. The levels of TMAO in the blood go up when we eat food high in L-carnitine or Choline. The food sources of L-carnitine are red meat and choline are, poultry, dairy, fish, and eggs. It is not a simple equation that when we eat these foods, the blood level of TMAO rises. There is another intermediate but essential step: the presence of certain specific types of bacteria in the intestines[212] that break down the L-carnitine and choline in the flesh and eggs and produce TMAO. The same person if they hold different types of (beneficial) bacteria in the intestine, then the TMAO levels don't rise after eating L-carnitine or Choline-containing foods. What determines whether the beneficial types or harmful types of intestinal bacteria build up in our system depends upon the meal pattern of the individual. In omnivores, exposure to animal foods changes the type of population in the gut bacteria to those that can increase TMAO when exposed to the L-carnitine and choline. In other words, eating animals changes the gut bacteria to the types that make it more dangerous to eat animals. How crazy is that? In humans who have been eating plant-based protein and other vegetables, fruit, nuts, seeds, and whole grains (essentially, all plant-based), their gut bacteria were found to change to the type that does not produce TMAO even after getting exposed to the meats or eggs. The study[213] that looked at it took a group of vegans and analyzed their blood levels of TMAO after they ate a piece of meat. The levels of TMAO remained flat. When the omnivore group ingested the same amount of meat, the levels of TMAO went up 6 times that of the plant-protein eaters. The mechanism of this is unclear, but scientists propose that the way the bacteria work to increase or decrease the risk of heart attack is by changing cholesterol traffic. Like the ABC proteins, these good bacteria keep the cholesterol traffic flowing away from the arteries into the gut excretion or into the liver as a second backup. In either situation, the traffic is nudged to move away from blocking the arteries and sent to leave the body when we have a bowel movement. When the cholesterol level in the bloodstream reaches a level that is beyond the capacity of our bowel clearance mechanism to get rid of this excess cholesterol, the body resorts to the second-rate option of packing the excess fats into the liver. In fact, this phenomenon transforms the liver into something we call "fatty liver."[214] Same as in Foie Gras, which is literally the fatty liver of a goose. One major difference is that in the case of the goose, it wasn't voluntarily eating the excess calories.[215,216]

J: My buddy Frank was told by his doc that he has a fatty liver!

B: It is not ideal to have that. Because it is a sign that there is excess cholesterol in the body, much more than what we need to make certain hormones. Essentially, we select the bacterial residents in our gut based on what we eat. Not consuming enough plant-based meals with adequate dietary fiber appears to facilitate settlers in the gut who are no good. They mess with the cholesterol traffic and lead to blocked arteries, meaning strokes and heart attacks. Eating such wholesome plant foods allows good bacteria to move into the gut neighborhood and keep the arteries clean from excessive cholesterol. Who would have known that billions of tiny buddies in our gut could decide the fate of whether or not we get a heart attack? These minions live in our gut. That is their home. What we eat directly goes to feed or hurt them, depending on what we choose to eat. It becomes super important to think about what we throw into their neighborhood using our forks, spoons, and knives.

J: You mean we shouldn't be regularly shoveling pieces of animals or processed food into our gut using our knives and forks the way we do now? Looks like that is not so gentle on the little buddies in our gut. The question is: is it too late for me to undo the damage?

B: Not according to Mrs. Reeves, who is now eighty-four years old.

J: Who's this person?

B: She and I went through a difficult illness when I was her body before she was eighty-four. Her heart was riddled with blockages, and one day, she and I felt the effects of her heart problems. She was out of breath, just from walking. The distance that she could walk before she had to stop to catch her breath became less and less. She went to see her doctor, who immediately sent her to a cardiologist. Testing showed that she had blocked coronaries, and what she was feeling as shortness of breath when she walked a few steps was angina related to poor oxygen flow from diseased arteries in her heart. Her cardiologist recommended that she get a heart bypass surgery because stenting the arteries were out of reach due to the way the arteries were blocked. She didn't want to. She went back to her primary care doctor, who recommended, as an alternative, to go on a whole-food, plant-based meal plan. She started eating this way at age eighty-four! In came a flood of nutrients from leafy greens, vegetables, fruit, wholegrains and flax seeds and a few walnuts and out went all animal foods, dairy, eggs, sugars, processed starches/snacks and virtually all cooking oil, yes even olive oil[217]. After a matter of two months, she is now able to walk for a few blocks, and she does not get shortness of breath. If she and others like her can reverse her blocked artery problem at age eighty-four, of course, you can at your age. I am built that way. On most instances, as long as you provide the right nourishment at the right dose, I can bounce back to reverse blocked heart arteries[218, 219, 220, 221, 222].

J: I still can't figure out something…

B: What's that?

J: What made this eighty-four-year-old woman make the changes in her food? I mean, I am not talking about her medical condition. What, in her essence, made it possible for her to shift her eighty-four-year-old behaviors. I know change can be hard, especially if you are used to a certain way of doing things for eighty-four years!

B: Her attitude. She was a stoic and gutsy woman. She had a great sense of humor. All she needed was motivation from the recent heart attack and the education that her doctor shared with her. When all these come together, anything is possible. Fundamentally, it starts with attitude.

J: But not everybody has that same attitude.

B: Not everyone has to continue with the same attitude. Attitudes can change.

J: How?

B: I believe it is about who we surround ourselves with in our lives. Some say that our interactions with the four people we spend most of our time in our lives determine our life's trajectory. They might be family members. Or, as one grows, he/she does have the freedom to choose the type of friends, neighbors, and partners in life and work to be with. Of the four people, one is inside of us. Our soul. Gut feeling, you may say. Others call it intuition. The ability to listen to this intelligence in you is fundamental. The message from this inner you has more clarity if we listen with an open mind without coloring the message with all our emotions, presumptions, and preset ideas about life and people. Are you cynical or optimistic? That can determine whether we can hear our intuition's message loud and clear. Another person among the four can come in the form of a mentor or a role model.

J: I get it now. The questions to think about are: Who do we hang out with most of our time in the day? Who are our mentors and role models? Are our minds open and uncolored by preset ideas or negative experiences in order to listen to our heart's message?

B: You got it. We do have control over making these choices of who we choose to be our mentors and role models. We do have control over clearing the clutter of preset ideas to look deeply and listen to what our heart says when it is not governed by fear or negativity.

J: I think I am ready.

B: For?

J: To make some changes in how I take care of myself.

B: I am all ears. Why would you want to do that?

J: I want to see my kids grow up and be there to witness their successes in life. I want to be active and energetic so that I can do the things I want to do in life. Currently, I can't do them because I just don't have the energy. Even if I try, my breathing gets harder, and I get tired easily.

B: I can tell from first-hand experience that when folks start to take care of themselves with proper sleep, good nourishment, and activity, I feel at my best while being part of them.

J: So, how do I start making some changes in my diet?

B: Well, it is actually very simple, and we can do it step by step. The first step would be to not skip your breakfast[223].

J: Really, I thought I was doing a good thing by skipping those calories. Of course, I am still not able to lose the extra body weight.

B: Skipping meals is part of the problem. You push me to work on alternative "famine physiology" when you skip meals[224]. I can't help but switch to that mode when you keep skipping meals.

J: What is "famine physiology'?

B: It is a mode I automatically switch to when I don't see calories coming in at a steady interval. In that mode, I anticipate "famine," and so in order to prepare for starvation, I save the calories from the next meal and store them. Also, a hormone called Ghrelin[225] gets released from the stomach to increase appetite to fix the famine.

J: Store them where?

B: In your belly and other fatty areas in the body. This way, they can be burned to be used when the starvation continues for many days.

J: But I don't starve for days. I just skip breakfast.

B: Correct. And that is when I switch to the alternate mode of calorie burning. I don't burn them all when you eat lunch and dinner that day. I store some of those calories as fat in the body. That is one of the reasons you cannot lose weight. In fact, research has shown that compared to people who eat breakfast on a regular basis, those men who skipped breakfast on a regular basis had a 27% higher risk of dying from heart attacks[226].

J: Wow, I never knew that. What should I include in the breakfast?

B: Whenever possible, fruit and vegetables. Combine 2-3 tablespoons of nuts with wholegrain breakfast. Some options are cooked oats or buckwheat or another type of wholegrain with some nuts and fruit. A teaspoon of raisins or dried fruit will help to sweeten it, if you wish. Using a savory breakfast with cooked vegetables and salsa or chutney with wholegrain wrap or flatbread is another option. Tofu scramble is a great substitute for egg scramble in the morning.

J: How much fruit should I eat in the morning?

B: At least one cup. That is a portion size of a tennis ball.

J: I always thought I should not eat fruit because it is all carbohydrates.

B: There are different types of carbohydrates. The good, healthy carbohydrate is the starch in fruit and vegetables, which have dietary fiber as well. There are some rare exceptions among fruit that can push up the sugar in your blood. Three fruits particularly come to mind: Pineapple, watermelon, and very ripe bananas.

J: I love those three fruits.

B: Yes, I know. It is interesting for me to notice that most of those I am part of who have a tendency for diabetes love these three fruits. It is almost like I can tell who among those I am part of will be getting diabetes down the line and who won't get into diabetes trouble based on their preference for these three fruits.

J: What about a banana that isn't very ripe?

B: That is fine. I feel happy when I see the meal on the plate has fruit with some seeds such as flax or sunflower or pumpkin seeds.

J: Why? What is with the seed combination?

B: The plant protein in the seeds slows down[227] how fast the glucose reaches to the peak level in the body. On the other hand, animal protein increases blood glucose[228] which leads to higher insulin levels that harm the arteries.

J: I am not getting it.

B: The risk of diabetes and injury to the lining of the arteries has a lot to do with how often and how much the bloodstream is flooded with insulin. The higher the insulin levels, the bigger the trouble is. The jump in insulin is preceded by a jump in blood sugar[229]. They go hand in hand. When the sugar level gets high in the blood quickly and quite often, it spells trouble through similar changes in insulin levels. The way to avoid this trouble would be to slow down how fast the glucose goes up in the blood from the starch in food and also how frequently that sugar hike happens. And that is where plant protein comes into play. If sugar is going on a high-speed highway, the protein in the meal acts like multiple speed bumps, thus slowing down the speed with which sugar goes up and down in the blood. So, combining plant protein like seeds or a tablespoon of nut butter with fruit keeps me happy.

J: What about other protein sources?

B: Plant protein protects me[230], so I prefer that in as many meals as possible. In savory dishes, it is great when someone combines protein, such as beans or lentils, with starch, such as wholesome rice or pasta.

J: I don't mind trying that combination. How often should I try this?

B: As often as possible. Initially, it will be great even if you experiment with just three plant-based protein dishes every week. In your case, because you just had a recent heart attack, I recommend moving from three dishes to more often quite quickly. Just one more thing, make sure that the dishes are not only healthy but tasty as well!

J: Believe me, I will make sure. If it ain't tasting good, it ain't going to last on my menu for long.

B: It is true. I also change my taste preference as you move away from eating some of the processed, unhealthy food.

J: How do you do that?

B: Well, for instance, if someone I am part of eats a lot of sugar and desserts, I automatically increase the bar for when I send a satisfactory signal for sweet taste to the brain. As a result, the next time that person takes something that has a little less sugar, it won't satisfy them[231]. They will end up eating more and more sugar until they burn most of the insulin in my pancreas (or theirs). The neat thing that I can do is when someone starts using wholesome food without sugar and processed starch, like white bread and cookies, I can lower the bar of the sweet taste threshold. So, after a few weeks or months of wholesome food, the carrot starts tasting sweet enough.

J: But if I am eating the carrot before you lower the sweet-tasting threshold?

B: That is when the carrot and broccoli might taste like cardboard.

J: I have been there when I attempted to eat healthy a few years ago.

B: I know. I was there, too.

J: Okay, what about protein?

B: Yes, I am glad you brought it up. First of all, I just need to get it out there. People are eating too much protein, much more than what they can handle. Rather, what I can handle. That is one of the first misconceptions I would like to talk about. The value given to what is needed for protein is mostly higher than what the true value is. So, we grow up believing that we need a ton of protein to become strong individuals when, in reality, we need a smaller amount of protein. Even a growing infant's entire diet, that is in mother's breast milk, protein contributes only 6%[232] of the calories. So, if we use 10% of calories coming from protein for example, a person who needs sixteen hundred calories daily needs only a minimum of forty grams of protein. In other words, in this person who needs sixteen hundred calories per day, if they have two meals for the day and don't get 10 grams of protein, then they are not getting enough protein for that day.

J: Twenty grams? That seems very low.

B: It is correct. For someone who needs two thousand calories a day, they need a minimum of fifty grams of protein only for the day. There are exceptions where the protein needs are a bit higher, as in teenagers growing up. Now, if this person is a professional athlete or bodybuilder, they may need extra protein - something in the range of sixty to seventy grams of protein.

J: How did you arrive at fifty grams for the two thousand calories per day? How does one know how many calories are needed for a day?

B: It is easy to calculate the caloric need these days with the availability of the internet. There are free calorie calculators available online[233]. A person would need a few basic details such as the current body weight, height, age, and level of physical activity. The calculator uses this information to tell how many calories someone needs to eat daily to maintain the weight that was entered for the calculation.

J: Oh, wait! What if that person is trying to lose weight and doesn't want to maintain that weight entered in the calculator?

B: It is easy. Just take away 400 calories from the calculated result and aim for that caloric intake to lose weight. So, for instance, if the number from the calculator says two thousand, then subtract four hundred, and you end up with sixteen hundred calories for the day to lose weight.

J: Interesting. That would mean they need even fewer grams of protein per day if it is sixteen hundred calories, not two-thousand. How does one calculate the grams of protein needed in daily diet from the value of daily caloric need?

B: It requires a bit of calculation. But I know you are numbers person, being an accountant and all.

J: Ha ha!

B: So, each gram of protein gives 4 calories. If a person needs sixteen hundred calories per day and ten percent of that total needs to come from protein, how many calories is that which needs to come from protein.

J: Easy. Remove a zero from sixteen hundred. We got one hundred and sixty.

B: Good. Now divide that one hundred and sixty by the 4 calories to arrive at how many grams of protein is required for the day.

J: Got it. Forty grams of protein. That is far fewer than what I originally assumed would be needed.

B: Correct. Protein need is routinely overestimated based on assumptions not objectively calculating the numbers.

J: So, it is all about the calories, isn't it?

B: Not quite. But we will come back to that later. Now, I am on a roll with this protein enlightenment, and let's keep going with that. The second misconception about protein that I want to address is that it is widely thought that animal protein is "superior" to plant protein for the body, for me. To be honest, that thinking is simply not true[234]. Plant protein has all the material that I want. I don't miss any amino acids as long the person is eating a variety of plant foods, like they should be, with fruit, vegetables, legumes, whole grains, nuts, and seeds[235, 236].

J: But what about building muscle?

B: No problem. I can use plant protein from beans, lentils, nuts, and seeds to build muscle.

J: What about energy? Doesn't plant protein give less energy than animal protein?

B: That is the third misconception I wanted to clear up. Thank you for bringing that up. When it comes to extracting energy from the food that comes at me, I have to work much harder to extract energy from protein – all proteins, plant or animal. It is much easier for me to pull energy from carbohydrates and fats to send it through the blood to the muscles and brain of someone who is working their mind and body. In other words, if you are going to physically exert yourself, it is easy for me to send the energy to you if you eat carbohydrates or a little bit of good fat before your physical activity. Have you heard of VO2 max?

J: What is it - a gym equipment?

B: Connected to physical activity indeed. It is a measure of the fitness of one's lungs and heart. If you are running a sprint contest toward the finish line, your VO2 max is the amount of oxygen consumed by your muscles when you are working your hardest to be the winner. The number is expressed as a milliliter of oxygen for every minute spent on every kilogram of your body weight. The fitter someone is, the higher this VO2 max number is. In fact, one study that compared women eating vegetarian diets with those eating omnivorous diets showed that not only did the vegetarian women show no weakness in this regard, but it also showed a slightly higher fitness of heart and lungs than the omnivorous group[237]. Another study[238] tested two groups of women - one eating omnivorous meals and the other fully plant-based meals. They were asked to pedal a stationary bicycle and maintain a set range of speed. The researchers were looking to see which group first reached the stage of exhaustion and which group could outlast the other. Contrary to popular belief, the group of women who were eating plant-protein, healthy carbohydrates such as vegetables, whole grains, and fruit were, on average, found to last three and half minutes longer than the omnivorous group could keep going with the pedaling of the bicycle.

J: That goes against what I believed. Why did the plant-eating bicycle women have more endurance?

B: The scientists who did the research believe that there was less inflammation in the plant-eating group, which assisted the muscles to keep going longer. Similarly, oxidative stress is thought to be less in plant-based eaters, which helps with muscle recovery. Additionally, carbohydrates are something I can use more efficiently to fuel the muscles[239].

J: I didn't know this about which nutrient gives energy easily. What carbohydrates are preferable?

B: Fruits and vegetables. If you are going to work hard and burn a lot of calories, then you may want to include vegetables that are grown below the ground, the root vegetables, because they are caloric dense.

J: Are potatoes okay?

B: Yes. Sweet potatoes have more nutrients, such as Vitamin A, than regular white potatoes, so I recommend mixing it up between different types of root vegetables before a workout.

J: What about whole grains? Nuts?

B: If you are going to work harder, adding whole grains such as rice or pasta before working out is fine. Nuts contain high calories, so anything more than a handful should be reserved for extreme athletes who burn a lot of calories on a regular basis.

J: What is a safe level of eating nuts at this stage of my life?

B: Since you got promoted to the management job, you are not physically exerting much at your workplace, so your routine practice is not suited to burn calories. Once you start taking up some routine physical activity, then I can handle the calories from eating nuts - just don't overdo it!

J: I am going to think about protein in a new light from now on. But don't we have to replace the protein that is broken down during hard workouts?

B: It is true. Timing is everything. So prior to working out, rely on starches, root vegetables, fruit, whole grains, and some nuts for good fats. After your workout, in order to rebuild muscle protein, eating protein-rich food is ideal. I recommend relying on beans, lentils, whole grains, nuts, or seeds for getting the necessary proteins. A variety of some of these plant foods will cover protein needs after working the muscles. And let's not forget that even green leafy vegetables, potatoes, and cabbage have some protein in them.

J: Great! I don't like the burning feeling that I get after working out my muscles.

B: Well, the burning you feel is unrelated to protein breakdown. It is related to the build-up of oxidant stress, which is like a 'bull in the China shop' breaking important structures inside the cell.

J: That sounds like trouble.

B: Correct. Oxidative stress is the reason behind the burning of muscles. So consuming colorful fruits and vegetables after working your muscles will help minimize the burning.

J: Neat. So, I will pack some green salad with chickpeas and nuts for a post-workout snack. Let's summarize our discussion.

---

1. Healthy lining of the arteries (endothelium) protects the heart.
2. ABC transporter proteins and cholesterol traffic mechanism keeps excess cholesterol out of the circulation to prevent blockage in arteries. Long-term inflammation impairs this traffic.
3. Excess junk food, processed food, excess fats and animal protein result in long-term inflammation and injures endothelium and plants the seed for artery blockage.
5. Secondary bile acid removes excess cholesterol through stools. Plant-foods rich in fiber facilitates this elimination.
5. Leafy greens, vegetables and fruit provide antioxidants that protect the weak spots in the lining of arteries.
6. Without dietary fiber and friendly gut bacteria, heart attack/stroke risk increases with high TMAO level in blood.
7. Wholefood, plant foods without oil can melt/dissolve blockages in heart's arteries.
8. VO2 max – high athletic performance with more plant foods.

CHAPTER FIVE
AGING: WHY THE RUSH TO AGE?

> Seven-word synopsis
> ***Healthy meals, relations & regular resting delay aging***

Body: Hello Grace!

Grace: I know you. What a long trip we have had together. I can't believe I am ninety-six. A lot of the people I meet can't believe that I am ninety-six.

B: That is because you garden for two hours every day, you take care of your house yourself, and nobody can forget how you put up the new raised bed for your garden last month. Most people are amazed and inspired by your strength, and a few are frankly annoyed by it. They don't know what to do with what they are seeing in your strength and vitality. Soon, they are going t conclude that you are doing some drugs to keep you going this strong!

G: That is very funny. I don't do drugs, nor do I take drugs prescribed long term. I have tried to do whatever I can not to break what is mine, including my health. That way, I can limit the need for long-term dependencies, such as prescription medications or a wheelchair.

B: Can we tell the world your ninety-six-year-strong secrets?

G: There isn't much to it. I just eat simple and tasty food that I have learned to prepare and share with others when listening to music and jokes. I keep active, and I laugh often.

B: They are going to want to know specifics about your food. Everyone is going to age. Some, like you, age late. How?

G: Well, my doctor once told me that one of the most important things to watch for is AGE.

B: What do you mean? We are, of course, talking about age and how you keep young at this age.

G: When I say A.G.E., I mean Advanced Glycated End-products. It was a mouthful for me when I learned it first from my doctor. When the blood levels of AGE are high in a person, guess what it does to her/him?

B: Wait, it ages them?

G: Yes, really quickly. If someone comes and asks me the opposite question, "What is the fastest way to age?" then I would suggest starting with eating fried and burnt food. These increase the A.G.E levels in the blood[240]. Then, to guarantee that they age really fast, they should stop eating enough colorful fruits and vegetables[241] and start eating more chicken, eggs, fish, meat, and dairy to increase inflammation in the body.

B: Wait, there are more than a few points you just told us about food. Let's break it down and go over them one at a time. Which fried food? What do you mean by burnt food?

G: Any fried food. Whether it is animal flesh or fresh vegetables, frying them in oil will increase the Advanced Glycated End-products in the blood after eating them. The change in the blood level of A.G.E. is worse with animal food than frying a potato, for instance.

B: You mean it happens with chips, French fries, and fried dough?

G: Yes, it happens with whatever you fry in oil.

B: But it tastes so good when you fry it, doesn't it?

G: Yes, for a fleeting moment, when it hits the tongue, it does taste good. It fires the signal for the pleasure /reward system in our brains and makes us feel good. The fat or oil is what gives that pleasure feeling. I learned that foods trigger our ancient dopamine/pleasure system in the brain simply for survival instincts. Why? That fat or oil is a great source of calories for survival in a world without food where we need to search for food. So, when calories are available in plenty, and we get exposed to high-calorie fats as in fried food, our system (taste buds and brain) are wired to pick out such high-calorie foods[242] because it will come in handy when life is all about searching for the next meal. But for those of us living in a privileged and industrialized world, we don't have to search in the forest for the next meal. We just need to open the fridge, drive, or walk to the store or restaurant on the corner of the street.

B: I am glad you stated this. I wish others would see this. I am the same body humans had 10,000 years ago when agriculture wasn't invented, and people had to forage for food. I find myself now in a sea of high-calorie, high fat, and highly processed food and find my pleasure/dopamine system is hyper-stimulated, and I don't have a stop switch for this primal instinct for seeking these foods once I get exposed to them. It is a big tease for me and whoever I am part of.

G: Yes, the best motivator for me was that I didn't want to be dependent on others, with rickety joints that wouldn't let me move around and take care of myself. I didn't want the burden of taking care of me to fall on my loved ones. By the way, the wrinkles I started developing on my skin inspired the final push of motivation. I wanted no more wrinkles. Out went the A.G.E.ing food from my diet[243,244].

B: Sure, that is a great motivator. What about burnt food? You mean grilling the food?

G: Not only grilling but any kind of heat that is too much and too long can burn the food. Whether it is food cooked directly over the flame, grilled, sautéed, or oven-baked.

B: So, are you talking about the black, charred areas in the food after cooking them?

G: Exactly. I say never eat them if you want to stay young.

B: You mentioned not eating enough fruit and vegetables as a problem. What has that got to do with aging?

G: See, the A.G.E. levels are just one of the problems. Everyday wear and tear in the body is another major problem.

B: Let's hear more about it! I want to see if that matches with what I have known about wear and tear. Most people don't understand that the rate of this wear and tear can be slowed down by proper care and maintenance of me, the body.

G: Most people do that for their cars, boats, motorbikes, and bicycles. You would think they would do the same for the body. Yes, the wear and tear in the cells in the body can definitely be slowed down by choosing to eat more colorful fruits and vegetables in our daily meals. The idea here is to flood our systems and blood circulation with anti-oxidants that are found in colorful fruits and vegetables. These anti-oxidants are 'anti', i.e., against the toxic build-up in the body's tissues due to everyday wear and tear.[245, 246] I don't want sewage building up in my system. That is what happens if we don't eat foods with anti-oxidants to do the cleanup. Who would want their house to have a toxic mess building up without a way to clean it?

B: How can people start cleaning up if they are not used to eating colorful fruits and vegetables?

G: Just start trying new foods. The way to wisdom for delaying aging is to try food that cleans up the oxidative stress and to avoid food that degenerates our joints, blocks our memory cells, carves wrinkle lines on the face, and paints our hair gray.

B: What if they don't like the new vegetables they try?

G: Well, how was it prepared? Some are good fresh, like grapes, carrots and tomatoes. Some need preparation with other vegetables, herbs, sauces, etc. Sometimes, it is a hit or miss when trying new things. Stopping to try at that point is a failure. Keeping up with trying new things in healthy food builds wisdom for caring for oneself to stay young.

B: Is it okay to cook the vegetables, or should they be eaten only raw, uncooked?

G: If possible, having a good portion of the food as fresh, uncooked vegetables, is good. When cooking, watching and ensuring the food is not overcooked and burnt is good. And, of course, frying in oil or eating charred /burnt parts of the meal is a fast track to arthritic joints, wrinkles, and gray hair. A.G.E. -

inducing foods and unmanaged stress partner together to age someone faster. On the highway of fast life, toxic food meets stress to practice transforming a youthful mind and body into a degenerate one as the clock keeps ticking in a rushed world. Every bump on an arthritic joint, every neuronal synapse in the brain that is empty of precious memories, and every wrinkle with twists and turns which arrived sooner rather than later has a story to tell about the opportunities to switch fried food or burnt meat to antioxidant rich wholefoods. They are choices showing up as contour lines changing the landscape of not only the joints, memory synapses, and facial skin but also the quality of life and longevity. I wanted to postpone those changes as long as possible.

B: Why did you mention chicken, eggs, meats, and dairy?

G: It has to do with inflammation. These foods increase inflammation in the body, which can, in turn, age the cells. The cells and tissues can't take it when they are hit from all directions, including inflammatory foods, fried and burnt food, and not having enough of a workforce in the form of antioxidants to clean up the oxidative stress, aka "wear and tear."

B: Right, oxidative stress. I know how it feels!

G: Most people feel it as cancer, arthritis, heart attacks, or infections due to poor immune systems.

B: Those are big ones! Can we totally avoid getting into this stress? I don't like the sound of how it can affect me.

G: It is hard to prevent this oxidative stress completely. Even if we live in a pristine environment without any pollution and clean water and air, it is still possible for someone living in such a place to build up some oxidative stress in their bodies—for instance, sleep. If someone living in that clean environment has problems with sleep due to stressful life events, that will build up oxidative stress. On top of this, there is a slow building up of this stress due to everyday wear and tear of cells in the body, purely as a by-product of just being.

B: Forget it. So, if someone living in a clean environment gets into this kind of trouble, imagine someone living in a polluted, highly developed city where they are exposed to all kinds of carcinogenic pollutants, continue to smoke, and live under high stress. That is a recipe for high oxidative stress load.

G: To make matters worse, imagine that this person or child dislikes eating colorful fruits and vegetables or they live in a food desert or food insecure situation where access to such fruit and vegetables is ridden with hurdles[247] due to the living environment where they can afford to live. Colorful fruits and vegetables provide antioxidants to counter the oxidant stress (also called oxidative stress or free radical injury).

B: It is like burning the candle on both ends. On one end, there is plenty of exposure to build up oxidative stress. On the other end, there is a lack of antioxidants to counter the effect of this oxidant damage.

G: Exactly. Then how do you expect people to age well?

B: So, to delay aging, we need to eat more fruit and vegetables, limit or stay away from inflammatory foods such as meats, eggs, and dairy, and avoid A.G.E.ing foods such as burnt or fried food. Frying food regularly is a fast track to aging.

G: Well said.

B: What else can people do besides nutrition strategies to delay aging?

G: Good sleep and meditation.

B: I know. It is amazing how much I can recharge the system when the person whom I am part of is sleeping, in hypnosis, or just meditating. I put my adrenaline system to rest. Sleep mode is recharge mode.

G: Yes, the more we can unwind the adrenaline system, the better it is for our system. Sleep, self-hypnosis, or meditation are the best tools for that. I get roughly seven hours of restful sleep.

B: It is a welcome break for me after going through a busy day with someone where the adrenaline system is constantly revved up and running. The scientific lingo for the adrenaline system is the sympathetic system. The opposite system, which is all about rest and relaxation, is called the parasympathetic system. Things that stimulate the rest and relaxation system are sleep, meditation, hypnosis, belly laughs, and belly breathing.

G: Belly breathing? And belly laughs?

B: Yes. Do you know about Vagus?

G: Las Vegas?

B: No, Vagus. V, A, G, U, S. It is a nerve in the body. One of the longest nerves in my nerve department. It likes traveling, like a vagabond, which is actually the reason it is called Vagus. It runs from the brain, through the neck, and into the abdomen and controls automatic functions of the heart, lungs, and intestines. In other words, what happens in Vagus doesn't stay in Vagus.

G: Ha ha!

B: Exactly, that belly laugh and similar belly breathing done in yoga are the ways to stimulate the Vagus nerve and create relaxation.[248] You see, in the body's set-up, this nerve needs to travel from the head through the neck and chest to the abdomen. There are many things in the way, like the diaphragm, the dome-shaped umbrella-like structure in between the chest and the abdomen. So, nature has provided gates through which things can travel from the chest to the abdomen and vice versa.

G: Like the holes that come with the old-style entertainment furniture for TV and video players. There were holes for the cable to go from the video player to the television.

B: Exactly. So, the gap in the diaphragm through which the Vagus passes through is the same as the passage for the food pipe (esophagus). So, you see, it is a crowded passage, and any significant movement of the diaphragm can stimulate the Vagus nerve to create the relaxation response. It is this kind of diaphragm movement that happens in belly breathing in yoga.

G: And belly laughs?

B: Yes. Laughter is key for relaxation[249]. The opposite is true, too. When we have our guard up it causes a stress reaction in the body. Imagine how many people are in relationships where they are stay silent, don't speak up or can't let their guard down. There is an epidemic of stress going on in the world. In your case, it is amazing how you are always surrounded by friends and other family members. Your energy is so positive and magnetic that they are drawn to you and spending time with you.

G: It is all good. I keep busy involving myself with community projects and contributing my skills in accounting as a volunteer in community organizations.

B: It is true. That sense you have of belonging in a community or a tribe, or however one wants to call it, improves health. It is a prescription for health[250, 251, 252, 253, 254, 255]. Can you imagine that this sense of belonging in a group can actually reduce inflammatory markers in the human blood[256]? So, it isn't just stress that is reduced but also inflammation! The opposite is true as well. A sense of loneliness is a strong influence in causing disease and death.[257] The same negative effect of isolation extends to the animals kept in captivity[258] as well, not just for humans.

G: Interesting!

B: It is true, whether it is human or non-human animals, all of us need to be part of a tribe, a community, or a network made of friends, like-minded individuals, or family. That is a prescription for health! Let me summarize what we shared in this conversation:

---

1. A.G.E. (Advanced Glycated End-products) and age increases with consuming fried and burnt foods
2. Oxidative stress accelerates aging. Antioxidant-rich leafy greens, fruit and vegetables neutralizes this stress.
3. Poor gut health from high-sugar, high-fat, low-fiber foods and visceral fat from excess calories contribute to long-term inflammation, which accelerates aging.
4. Sleep, relaxation, and mindfulness approaches stimulate the vagus / noradrenaline system to recharge the body.
5. Staying active is key to delaying aging.
6. Having social connections with healthy relationships and finding and belonging in a community literally saves lives.
7. Purpose in life is a pill for staying young.

CHAPTER SIX
THE SIXTH SENSE ORGAN: GUT FEELING

> Seven-word synopsis
> ***Fibrous, unprocessed plant foods heal gut inflammation***

Jen: This is definitely a better feeling. Different from the constant waves of anxiety and the deep pit of emptiness I was feeling in my stomach. Who are you? And how did you end up chatting with me? I thought I was doing the meditation that my therapist had been recommending for many months for my anxiety and depression.

B: I am your body. You are in a kind of trance[259] that not everyone gets into during meditation, but it can happen. It is just temporary. It is a safe space to chat.

Jen: Okay, this is strange! Well, if you are my body, then perhaps you can clarify some things I am wondering about.

B: Sure thing. Go ahead.

Jen: My therapist tells me that the way I am feeling in my head space is related to my gut. That I am feeling anxious and depressed due to my gut problems.

B: Correct. It is not surprising that someone can feel anxious or depressed if maintaining a social life is made difficult by gut problems. You had been having to think twice before accepting any party invitations and had to avoid such events if they were longer than an hour or involved large groups. It was messing with your ability to be yourself in any social situation. That is bound to have an effect on your mood. It is understandable that you feel the way you do.

J: Yup. That's similar to what my therapist said. She gave me a few resources, including this reference for mindfulness meditation. I was desperate to feel better, so I gave it a try because this opportunity landed on my lap during this weekend trip. And, here I am talking to myself, a good kind of 'talking to myself,' I guess.

B: I was an integral part of your journey right from the early stages when you started to have intestinal issues. Right from high school. I tried to send you messages to seek assistance before it got to the next stage of illness.

J: It looks like I might have ignored your early signals. But I am glad that at least I am seeking assistance now.

B: Absolutely. It is still early in the course of your Crohn's disease, so the good thing is that it isn't too late to make changes in your lifestyle to mitigate the issue and avoid complications from the illness.

J: We will see! I am listening in order to learn and give it a shot in changing my lifestyle. Not socializing is depressing and thinking about meeting people outside my home makes me sick to the stomach. It is awful that this illness gets you in your teenage years.

B: Yes, unfortunately, one in four individuals who get Crohn's disease or Ulcerative Colitis develop the disease before they reach age 20.[260] These two illnesses are both grouped into the 'Inflammatory Bowel Disease' category in the medical world and more and more people are getting this problem[261].

J: How is Ulcerative Colitis different from what I got? My physician told me that there was inflammation in my gut.

B: Which part of the gut is involved can vary between what you have, which is Crohn's disease, and what others have when diagnosed with Ulcerative Colitis. Ulcerative Colitis affects only the large intestine ('colon + itis' where the 'itis' implies inflammation as in 'arthritis').

Crohn's disease can affect any location in the gut, starting from the mouth, throat, and food pipe ('esophagus') all the way to the rectum and anus.

However, the common signature in both conditions is inflammation[262], which is the equivalent of wildfire in the gut. This inflammation doesn't happen by itself, much like most wildfire doesn't start spontaneously out of nowhere. Yes, a genetic influence[263] runs in the family for these two bowel diseases - more so for Crohn's disease than Ulcerative Colitis. However, just because someone has the gene transferred from the parent to her/him doesn't mean that she/he is going to develop the disease ("epigenetics")[264] - much like just because there are dry leaves and dead plants on the floor of the forests doesn't mean that they are going to catch fire. Other things need to come together in that tinderbox for the fire to start, such as the lack of moisture in the soil due to lack of rain and extremely hot weather. Again, much like the lack of friendly bacteria in the gut that would have cooled down the inflammation ('heat') in the gut lining. Of course, there is a human element for wildfires, with 80% of wildfires caused by human behavior, such as smoking a cigarette and throwing it on the forest floor. Likewise, a very common influencer of inflammatory bowel disease is human behavior, in this case mostly done inadvertently, by choice of meals when growing up and into adulthood. Meaning a diet lacking in dietary fiber necessary to build friendly gut bacteria. That is the equivalent of moisture in the soil in our wildfire analogy to cool down the risk of fire and inflammation from happening.

J: My mom told me that my grandmother had long-term bowel issues. I am pretty sure that I have the genes for it. You said that I could change something in my lifestyle to mitigate the illness. How do we know that it is not mainly due to the family's genetics? I have heard people say that we couldn't do anything about preventing Crohn's or Ulcerative Colitis.

B: Genetics do play a small role, but as I just said, there are other conditions and instigators that override the genes and determine whether the fire is going to be 'ignited'.

When researchers studied the connection between family genes that carry the risk for inflammatory bowel diseases and the true development of those diseases, they found evidence that genes are not in the driving seat to take that person to that unfortunate disease destination. To a large degree, the individual has control over the destination if they choose to. For instance, twins who carry the exact carbon copy of genes, including genetic risk for inflammatory bowel diseases, don't manifest the disease equally when they grow into two adults[265] - what researchers call the 'concordance rate' in twins. One hundred percent concordance means the health outcomes are one hundred percent similar in both twins with exactly similar copies of genes. If this number is less, then it means that one twin didn't get the disease even after bearing the same risky gene. For Crohn's, the disease concordance rate is around fifty-eight percent. That means in the remaining forty-two percent of the twins who carried the genetic risk for Inflammatory Bowel Disease, one of the pairs didn't develop the disease in their adult life. The concordance rate for Ulcerative Colitis is even less. In more than 90 percent of the twin pairs carrying the genetic risk, one of the pairs did not develop the disease, meaning the influence of genes was minimal to none. So, factors other than genetic risk matter a lot[266].

Jen: Okay, I can't blame grandma as much for this, I guess.

B: There's more data to support this concept. The prevalence of Inflammatory Bowel Diseases has been increasing over the past 50 years; too fast of a change to blame it all on changes in human genetics[267], which (the latter) can take millions of years. Lifestyle and exposure to different triggers[268] in food behaviors over the past fifty to sixty years can explain the rapid increase in prevalence that genetics cannot explain.

Additionally, children of those who immigrate from developing countries to Western countries show rates of Inflammatory Bowel Disease occurrence similar to that of Western populations compared with their family members of the same age who stayed back in their native country with the native food and lifestyle[269]. Same genes, different exposure to risks, and different outcomes[270]. Genes getting outdone by lifestyle again.

Jen: So what was going on in the bodies of twin sisters and twin brothers who dodged the disease through a better lifestyle?

B: Well, one fundamental thing they did is to balance the levels of healthy and harmful bacteria in the gut to tip toward more healthy bacteria[271]. The main strategy to achieve this[272] is by adding more meals that are high in dietary fiber[273, 274, 275, 276, 277] such as leafy greens, vegetables, legumes, and fruits, and by switching grains and grain-based food to whole grains, as in switching to whole grain pasta or bread or unprocessed rice or other grains.

This better balance in the bacterial population fixes two other malfunctions that allow for these two diseases to develop into full-blown illnesses:

1. Break in the protective fence[278, 279] along the inner lining of the gut

2. Breakdown in the immune function housed in the gut

J: Tell me about the fence first.

B: This defense barrier is called the 'mucosal barrier[280, 281]' by the science folks. Basically, it is the lining of the gut that puts up a strong barricade against many unwanted chemical and biological materials in the food we consume and prevents them from entering into our blood stream or getting picked up by the radar of our immune defense system. When this barrier fails, a large number of microorganisms (bacteria, viruses, etc.) are no longer insulated from the immune system housed in the gut and come in direct contact with the immune cells, triggering excessive force as a response from the immune system. Why would you use a fire hose to remove weeds in the garden? Such a strong return fire, when recurrent, results in long-term inflammation of the gut, setting the stage for Crohn's and Ulcerative Colitis.

Simply put, if the barrier is strong, no alarm bells or triggers are going on in the immune system and hence no return fire, and as a result, all is cool and well in the gut.

This fence that insulates the immune system from getting riled up is built with five layers of defense:

The mucosa layer is the sticky gel-like coat /lining of the intestinal tube that comes directly in contact with the contents of the intestine. This gel layer is not a physical barricade but also has antibiotic-like abilities to neutralize harmful microbugs.

Making up the second layer are fighter molecules embedded below the sticky gel layer. Two types of these molecules are notable: Antimicrobial protein-chains (aka 'peptides') and antibodies also known as Immunoglobulin A.

The third layer is a physical shield made of cells tightly stitched together to form a strong barrier called 'Epithelium.'

Beneath this, the fourth layer is a wall with fighter cells embedded in the wall ("Lamina propria"), a layer chock full of cells that release antibodies, white blood cells that can eat up harmful bacteria, and T immune cells that have long term memory of unwelcome microorganisms that come through food and fluids consumed.

The final and the most valuable player in the defense line-up is formed by the friendly bacteria of the gut. They reinforce the other four layers of this formidable defense barrier in the sense that they are like the captain of the team of five layers trying to insulate the immune system from getting exposed to triggers in the gut tube. The weakness of the friendly bacteria, for instance, when they are not fed with dietary fiber and are starving, leads to weakening the entire five layers of the fence[282, 283]. In other words, what is on the meal plate, more specifically, how much of the meals have dietary fiber, is key to defending against exposure to unwelcome stimulations that trigger unnecessary and excessive immune response, which leads to long-term inflammation of the gut tube.

J: So what happened to my five-layer fence?

B: Your friendly bacteria were weak without being fed with enough dietary fiber, so they couldn't keep the five layers strongly held together[284]. The third layer, 'Epithelium,' started to show gaps, making it essentially porous, letting in unwelcome guests[285, 286] through the fence to places where they don't belong - next to the immune cells. Of course, your immune cells reacted with heavy return fire. Also, your natural antibiotic protein-chains ('Antimicrobial Peptides' shortly 'AMP'[287]) were too weak to stop the entry of microorganisms. The production machinery that recycles cell material to make more defense players in the sticky gel layer wasn't working well so that also resulted in more breaches and more return fire from your immune system. In order to fix these broken areas, your gut needed 'short-chain fatty acids' - something that the friendly bacteria makes out of dietary fiber[288, 289, 290, 291, 292, 293, 294], especially from leafy greens and beans[295]. Without enough supply of these foods in your diet, this fix was scarce to prevent inflammation from taking over in the small intestines.

J: Can I add more dietary fiber to my diet now to fix the problem?

B: You can, as long as you are not going through a flare-up of Crohn's. Best to start low and go slow in adding the dietary fiber when things are quiet with your Crohn's. When I say start low, what I mean is to not start right away with big portions of raw vegetable salads but rather with an incremental increase of cooked vegetables and beans when introducing dietary fiber. Every month, the dietary fiber portion can be increased over the course of the next few months to a tolerable level. This approach increases the chances of rebuilding the fence, stopping intrusion, and thus preventing the immune system from firing excessively[296].

Jen: You just reminded me of the immune system you mentioned earlier as a player in my gut inflammation. Tell me more about the disorder in immune function housed in the gut.

B: Our immune system guards us throughout our lives. The Immune cells are housed mostly in our gut and lymph-node-related organs, from where the lymph cells are released into the blood stream to provide defense. Immune cells reside all the way from our mouth to the small intestines. More are located in organs such as the spleen, thymus, lymph nodes, and lymph channels, bone marrow, outer skin and inner lining of the mouth, nostrils, wind pipes in lungs, and the lining of the urinary bladder and urethra. I usually compare the lymph nodes of a region to the town police station. Any trouble in the region will activate the police station of our immune system - the lymph nodes. So, if someone has a sore throat, the lymph nodes in the neck may become bigger and painful. That means the police station is busy working to catch the invading bugs. Stress and unhealthy food choices affect our immune system.

When I say stress, I mean physical and emotional stress. Things like staying up all night and being sleep-deprived. Long term emotional stress, major injuries etc.

More importantly, anything that affects the intestinal tract's health through coloring agents, junk food, and food additives can all affect the health of the friendly bacteria in the gut. The friendly bacteria are fundamentally important for the health of the gut. They depend on a nutrient-rich environment and our dietary fiber to sustain themselves. When we don't consume enough vegetables, leafy greens, beans, and fruit, food groups rich in dietary fiber, then we are essentially not feeding the good bacteria. When the good bacteria can't thrive well, intestinal health takes a big hit. We know that more than 60% of the immune cells are housed in the gut and its related organs. So, when we don't have healthy bacteria in the gut, we don't have a healthy immune system[297]. The immune system's strength is only as good as the diversity and strength of the friendly bacteria population in our intestines[298, 299, 300]. And the strength of the immune system is not all about its fire power but rather its ability to pull punches and not over-react in response to an insult or triggering event, as well as its ability, when needed, to bring its force to nuanced action that tackles the unwelcome guests while not attacking one's own organs. Such a calibrated response is the norm for a healthy immune system.

J: How does the healthy immune system manage to finely control its response?

B: In a healthy immune system, which is determined by a healthy gut environment with the right amount of friendly bacteria, there are controls in place to keep the immune system from over-reacting and to pull its punches. It is about striking the right balance between push and pull. The push is the force of immune attack as in the T-helper 17 cells[301] (for short, "Th-17"), which deal with unwelcome microorganisms entering our bodies. The pull is the control to avoid over-reaction by pulling the punches, the 'T-regulatory cells, or 'Tregs' for short. With the right balance of actions of Th-17/ Tregs, we have 'homeostasis[302, 303], the steady state of balance between two opposing actions, an ideal place for me.

Cells called 'Regulatory T cells', nicknamed 'Tregs[304],' do this job of controlling any over-reaction by the immune firepower by listening to a higher gatekeeper. Who sends these 'Tregs' to communicate the "hold the fire!" message to the immune system? The duo of friendly gut bacteria[305,306] and dietary fiber[307, 308]. When someone makes sure they eat leafy greens and beans regularly, these friendly bacteria break down the starchy fiber to produce short-chain fatty acids called 'Butyrates' which become messengers that signal to the 'Tregs'[309] to communicate to the immune system to hold the fire. Keeping the immune system in check from over-reacting is key to preventing long-term inflammation in the gut as well as other groups of imbalances called 'auto-immune diseases'. As you can imagine, when there are not enough leafy greens and beans in your diet, there are not enough of the 'Butyrate' messengers[310] to send 'Tregs' to rein in the immune system's fire when nuisance microorganisms breach the gut lining fence and rile up the immune system.

J: 'Butyrate' appears to be a key messenger.

B: Yes, I call 'Butyrate' the 'Super-Derivative' because of its superpowers even though it is a by-product of the breakdown of starch by friendly bacteria. For instance, Butyrate is the main source of fuel for the colon cells[311]. Without Butyrate production, colon cells will not be healthy[312]. An unhealthy colon cell has poor defense against cancer or inflammation and can easily turn into a colon cancer cell[313] or get inflamed long-term ('colitis'[314]). Having enough dietary fiber is the main strategy in fixing a meal to protect your colon. I knew this before but the science is catching up and understanding how beans and their breakdown products in the colon are acted upon by the colon bacteria to produce beneficial effects of preventing colon cancer[315, 316]. The action of the colon bacteria ferments the non-digested fiber of beans in the colon. These fermentation products work on the colon cells to stop the cancer growth by intervening in multiple mechanisms of colon cancer formation. Studies using colon cancer cells called HT-29 cells have confirmed[317] this finding of how this 'super-derivative' byproduct of beans consumed ('Butyrate') can interact with the colonic bacteria to stop colon cancers.

It appears that the beans and their super-derivative Butyrate prevent colon cancers by promoting normal colon cell maturation, by slowing down the rate of colon cell replication, and by selectively killing off any colon cells that assume cancer features of uncontrolled replication. Therefore, a greater increase in Short-Chain Fatty Acids (SCFA) production and potentially a greater delivery of SCFA, specifically Butyrate, to the colon may result in a protective effect on your colon. And leafy greens and beans can be the secret recipe for achieving this.

Propionate and Acetate are two other short-chain fatty acids produced in the intestines by the breakdown of starchy fiber by the bacteria.

The fatty acid Propionate has been shown to slow down excess production of cholesterol in the body.

J: My goodness. These short-chain fatty acids are slaying it! My friend who works at a coffee shop told me that she has Ulcerative Colitis. Will this dietary fiber also apply to his situation?

B: Correct. Except for some minor differences in the location of the problem, the issues and solutions are very similar for you and Joe's dad.

Jen: Can you summarize the most important elements of a dietary approach one needs to take to protect against Crohn's disease and Ulcerative colitis?

B: Let me summarize the most important elements using the MOST as an acronym.

Microbiome: Healthy gut bacterial balance

Optimize caloric intake: Adequacy of calories and macronutrients, namely carbohydrates, protein and fats.

Superior nutrition quality: Maximize quality of nutrition

Trigger foods: Minimize or avoid trigger food

M: The first M standing for Microbiome, refers to having a healthy balance of gut bacteria with plenty of friendly ones. It is first and fundamental to the other elements.

O: When going through any dietary change, it is important to make sure one is not reducing the caloric intake to unhealthy levels. Hence, **o**ptimal intake of adequate calories but not excessive calories is key to long-term health while navigating Crohn's or Ulcerative Colitis. **O**ptimal caloric intake also checks the box of making sure that the daily caloric intake supplies the minimum daily requirement of protein, starch to feed the brain, fiber, and healthy fats such as omega-3 fatty acids (called 'macronutrients').

S: Of course, taking just adequate calories and meeting the daily minimum macronutrient requirement is not enough. It is important to make sure that for every calorie we take, we get some bonus in the form of micronutrients such as vitamins, antioxidants, phyto-nutrients etc., that come along with the calories. That's superior nutrition with a capital S.

T: And, last but not least, all this good work doing MOS will be undone if not taking care of avoiding the T, the trigger foods that can pour fuel onto the fire of inflammation in the gut. The International Organization for Inflammatory Bowel Diseases recommends[318] to avoid or:

- Reduce consumption of red meat (beef, pork, lamb, deli meats etc.)
- Reduce consumption of myristic acid (palm oil, coconut oil, dairy fats)
- Reduce consumption of saturated fats
- Reduce the intake of emulsifiers and thickeners (e.g. carrageenan)
- and processed foods containing titanium dioxide and sulfites.
- Avoid trans fats, aka hydrogenated oils or partially hydrogenated oils
- Limit intake of foods containing maltodextrin and artificial sweeteners

As I mentioned earlier, the fundamental step is building the right balance of healthy microbiome in the gut with enough friendly bacteria.

Jen: Can't we just take probiotic capsules to improve the friendly bacteria count and then keep doing whatever we want to do without worrying about the effect on gut health?

B: No. It doesn't work like that.

The idea of taking probiotics is like seeding your garden. Just sowing the seeds alone is not going to create a wonderful garden. The patch of soil needs to have the right conditions for the seeds to grow – sunlight, water and the correct amount of nutrients and, guess what, a good amount of microorganisms in the soil to transport the nutrients to the growing seeds.

Would the garden grow if we seed the soil and do all kinds of toxic things without feeding them with water and sunlight? It won't. The same way, just taking the probiotic pills without feeding them with dietary fiber (from vegetables, fruit, whole grains, legumes) will lead to the death of probiotic seeds planted into the gut through the expensive bottle of capsules one buys.

So, what is the role of probiotic supplements?

B: The role of probiotics is limited to short term only and for certain periods in our lives. Taking them year-round is like seeding the soil year-round. Seeding is done at a certain time of the year, and then, more importantly, the right conditions for the seeds to grow are to be nurtured throughout the year (such as eating good amounts of dietary fiber and avoiding toxic additives and coloring agents and pesticide-laden food).

Jen: What if I don't want to take probiotics? Is there a way to manage having a good bacterial population in the gut without having to take probiotics?

B: The best way to get nutrients to improve long-term health usually is through whole, unprocessed foods and not pills or supplements. Yes, eating foods that are fermented and high in fiber can help with improving a good bacterial population. These are sometimes referred to as prebiotic foods[319, 320]. Examples would include the cruciferous group, such as broccoli, cauliflower, kale, and bok choy. Other vegetables, such as sauerkraut, Jerusalem artichokes, and fermented tofu (tempeh) are also prebiotics. And blueberries, peaches, apples, and green bananas are also good sources. And, of course, any vegetable or fruit high in dietary fiber is useful to promote a good bacterial population in the gut.

J: It is incredible that a healthy bacterial population well-fed with adequate dietary fiber can have such a positive effect on the entire gut system and the immune system housed in the gut.

B: It is beyond incredible when we realize the far-reaching effects of the gut microbiome on organs in the body far from the gut. It is like the healthy bacteria have a very tiny remote control which they handle using their micro 'hands'! The gut as an organ has highly sensitive sensory radars in the 'mucosal barrier' fence layers and in the ability of the microbiome to sense nutrients and calories coming in through the intestines. In that sense, the gut with its microbiome is the ***organ of the sixth sense*** in the line of organs we have for other senses, such as vision, hearing, taste, touch, and smell.

J: Wow! Far and beyond the gut? Tell me more about it.

B: Hmmmm......where do I start? Let's first start with calories and obesity. How we absorb the calories in our food and how our body utilizes these calories are determined by the intestinal bacteria[321]. Most of the carbohydrates and protein we consume and all of the fats we consume are absorbed by the time the food (or what is left) reaches the end of the small intestine and the beginning of the colon. Between ten and twenty percent? Of the total calories ingested are not absorbed until they reach the colon.

These calories are from carbohydrates (undigested fiber) and protein that wasn't absorbed upstream in the small intestines. The problem is that the cells of the colon (large intestine) are not good at the job of breaking down and absorbing nutrients. That job is best done by the small intestines. So, the helpless colon really needs assistance in breaking down the undigested fiber and protein to harvest energy (calories). The friendly bacteria in the colon are the champions that assist the colon by providing digesting enzymes that can break down this part of the food in the colon. For instance, to break down the starch fiber in the colon, we need an enzyme called glycoside hydrolase. Well, the human genetic system has 98 of these enzymes, which is really not enough to do the job. The colon bacteria *Bacteroides thetaiotaomicron* (*B theta*) provides 226 glycoside hydrolases [322, 323] and, as a bonus, gives 15 polysaccharide lyases (another group of enzymes to break down starch fiber). Vitally, there is a super-derivative produced when the bacterial enzymes break down the Fiber: Butyrate.

Friendly bacteria use butyrate to regulate the gut hormone secretions, thus controlling cravings, regulating the on and off switch for appetite, and consequently absorption of calories.

Additionally, the friendly bacteria also convert the liver-produced bile acid into 'bile acids 2.0' (science calls them 'secondary bile acids'). These 'bile acids 2.0' work to control energy expenditure, glucose and cholesterol in the body. So, essentially, maintaining a healthy level of friendly bacteria through dietary fiber can control excess weight, blood sugar, and blood cholesterol through the production of butyrate and 'bile acids 2.0'.

J: If the microbiome and a healthy gut can regulate excess cholesterol, then it sounds like the microbiome and gut health can actually help prevent heart attacks, too.

B: Correct.

Gut bacterial health and diversity have been implicated in other problems such as obesity, diabetes, pre-diabetes, nonalcoholic fatty liver disease[324], colon cancer, biliary diseases[325], circulatory disturbance, asthma[326], and allergic diseases[327].

B: There is much to be learned in this new emerging field of understanding how the gut bacterial genes influence health and disease. Basic things such as a healthy bowel movement and its regularity are all reliable signs of healthy gut bacteria, which in turn can determine good health, locally in the gut and systemically in the body elsewhere.

J: Wow! That's a lot of systems in the body that are affected by the bacteria in our intestines.

B: Newer evidence is also pointing to the concept of how gut bacterial health can be associated with autoimmune diseases. Before we go there, let me summarize what we discussed:

> 1. Gut lining ('mucosal barrier function") is vital to prevent gut inflammation.
> 2. Low-sugar, low-fat, high-fiber diet maintains gut health. This benefit is present even if there is a familial/genetic risk for Crohn's diseases or Ulcerative colitis.
> 3. People with inflammatory bowel disease will benefit from **MOST** approach to diet:
> **M**icrobiome: Healthy gut bacterial balance
> **O**ptimize caloric intake: Adequacy of calories and macronutrients, namely carbohydrates, protein and fats.
> **S**uperior nutrition quality: Maximize quality of nutrition.
> **T**rigger foods: Minimize or avoid trigger foods.

CHAPTER SEVEN
IDENTITY CRISIS: AUTOIMMUNE DISEASES

> Seven-word synopsis
> *Plant foods deploy 'T-regs', blocking autoimmune attacks*

Vulcan is known as the ancient Roman god of fire and metalworks. He is said to have been born to Zeus and Juno. Zeus, the king of Roman gods, ruled from Mount Olympus. When born, baby Vulcan was perceived by Juno as ugly looking, so she threw him down Mount Etna[328]. Baby Vulcan went tumbling down the mountain and ended up at the bottom of the ocean, where Thetis adopted him and raised him in her underwater world.

Growing up in the water world, one fine day, Vulcan finds a fisherman's fire and gets fascinated by a lump of burning coal, which he carefully locks into a clamshell and brings underwater to his ocean abode. On day two, he learns that if he made the fire hotter by using bellows to blow air, he could make certain stones sweat gold, silver, and iron. The next day, he learns to make ornaments with gold, silver, and iron. Vulcan was worshiped for his capacity for creating fire but was also feared for turning it into a destructive fire. On the one hand, his fire was considered as aiding in defense that prevented evil influences. On the other hand, it was feared that the fire's effects might turn inward and become self-destructive. As in ancient Roman and Greek mythology, the Vedic tradition from ancient India also speaks of the fire of defense used to avert evil influences. The Vedic writings describe Agni, the

Hindu god of fire[329], as having two faces - one benevolent and the other of wrath. The power of Vulcan's defense fire or Agni's benevolent fire can be analogous to the power of the innate fire power that our bodies can generate to defend against harmful pathogens such as bacteria and viruses. This fire in our bodies is called the immune system.

Now, do we need to fear the destructive power of our immune system like the ancient Romans feared the destructive power of the fire god Vulcan? Usually, we don't have to because we have controls in place to prevent the over-reaction of the immune system. In a rare event, we unfortunately end up suffering the wrath of our own immunity. Medical science calls it 'auto-immune disease,' where the word 'auto' is the word-forming element meaning 'by oneself,' which in turn is derived from the Greek word 'autos[330],' reflexive pronoun for "self, same." A name that is fitting for a self-destructive disease where one's own immunity attacks one's own native tissues and destroys them. What does this damage look like in the real world? The tragic manifestations of this self-destruction looks like a ten year old having to take insulin injections due to type 1 diabetes, where this "fire" destroys the pancreas cells that make insulin. It can look like rheumatoid arthritis with crippling joint pain and stiffness that makes simple tasks like opening a jar a monumental task. It can look like multiple sclerosis, bringing down a lively, energetic young person to becoming stuck in a wheelchair to move from one room to the next. In autoimmune diseases, the fire of immunity attacks the body's own tissues (as in 'friendly fire' in military terms), such as the pancreas, joints, brain, liver, adrenal glands, thyroid gland, eyes, kidneys etc.

What triggers the immune system to go haywire and start this relentless attack, not knowing the difference between friend or foe within the body's internal landscape?

Let's meet Lauren while she is learning, from listening to her body talk about her rheumatoid arthritis.

Lauren: Hello!

Body: Hello, I am your body. I am thrilled that we get to talk. I have been wanting to for a while.

Lauren: Strange. I won't shut you out. I have learned to listen to my gut ever since I learned to control my joint pain by eating differently. I am all ears!

B: Great! How about we start with fundamentals? Do you want to hear more about why people get 'auto-immune diseases'?

Lauren: Yes, especially how my family genes are connected or not connected to getting the disease.

B: That is a good place to start. It is more about nurture (how we treat our bodies) than nature[331, 332, 333, 334, 335, 336], that is the genes we are born with. What the body gets exposed to, especially diet[337, 338, 339, 340, 341] and antibiotics, and how that shapes the bacterial balance in the gut plays a key role in the development of auto-immune diseases[342, 343, 344, 345, 346].

L: Can you break it down for me?

B: Essentially, there are two steps that need to occur for the disease to begin. First, the immune system gets spooked and goes into hyper-alert when it comes 'face to face' with an unfamiliar entity. It realizes that an unwelcome guest is around and gets ready with what it is built to do - getting armed and looking to fire away the next time it recognizes that same 'face' of this unknown entity[347, 348].

Secondly, the regulatory control that usually reins in the firepower of the immune system doesn't work well, so the firing is unchecked, and excessive force is used, resulting in damage to one's own organs.

L: But why did the wrong, innocent target (a part of ourselves) come under such excessive force of fire?

B: Because of an identical match of the 'face.' Enter the world of molecular mimicry[349, 350, 351, 352, 353] to understand this fully. Yes, molecules mimic each other.

L: Which molecules? How is this connected with the friendly fire of autoimmune diseases?

B: Let's look at an analogy to explain this. Imagine a theft or a homicide in a neighborhood. What do the police do when they talk to a witness? They sketch the face of the suspect using the description given by the witness. The sketch is shared with other law enforcement departments everywhere in the region, sometimes in the whole country or even internationally when it involves international crimes. When the police see someone matching the sketch, they chase after that person. The same thing happens in molecular mimicry, starting a friendly fire. One molecule gets exposed to the immune system as an 'invading,' unwelcome foreign molecule because the body is not used to seeing it as native to one's own organs. Milk protein, for example. It is not native to the human body (remember, it is cow's milk). The body triggers a response when exposed to this foreign protein[354]. A sketch is drawn up by the immune cells and shared with the body's entire immune system. Anything that matches the sketch will be attacked. What if milk protein's molecular sketch mimics our own pancreas cells[355]? More precisely, the cells that produce insulin. Our immune fire will destroy those pancreas cells because they are just following the orders to go after whatever matches the identity on the sketch of the suspect. Now we have type 1 diabetes in 9 or 10 year olds because the insulin-producing cells are destroyed by friendly fire that mistook pancreas cells for the molecules of milk protein that mimicked the pancreas cells[356,357,358,359,360]. Even though the genetic tendency for this phenomenon is important, the genetic fuse is not lit until exposure to milk protein occurs in the child with that genetic tendency.

The longer the immune fire keeps raging, the more advanced is the type-1 diabetes stage. There won't be enough insulin-producing cells left in the pancreas to make insulin. In an advanced stage, the child will unfortunately end up being on insulin injections for life. Any child or parent who is going through the hardship of insulin shots and never-ending needle-pricks in the tip of the fingers to test blood sugar would be looking for a solution that can minimize this hardship. Today's technological innovations have made it possible for new medical devices that can continuously monitor blood sugar levels without having to stick needles in the fingertips multiple times on a daily basis. However, nothing can beat the ability to prevent Type 1 diabetes from happening in the first place.

L: Is it even possible to prevent type 1 diabetes in someone with a genetic tendency for it?

B: Yes. Getting type 1 diabetes is not a destiny written in stone by the twisted helix of genetic code carrying this disease gene to the child from the parents. The gene coding for type 1 diabetes by itself cannot manifest as the disease in a child[361] unless the child gets exposed to cow's milk protein[362]. The gene and dairy protein are two sides of this bad coin. In other words, exposure to cow's milk protein is essential for the gene to start the fire that destroys insulin-producing cells. Cow's milk protein can get in the child's stomach after weaning from breast milk in the form of cow's milk, cheese, yogurt, or butter.

This means that a child who is weaned off mother's milk and then switched to solid food without getting exposed to cow's milk is less likely to get type 1 diabetes. Even if the child has the gene for type 1 diabetes! Organic soy-based milk or baby formula is a reasonable alternative[363]. It is also worth noting that a specialized baby formula made by breaking down the cow's milk protein through a chemical process ('hydrolysis') may not trigger the autoimmunity[364] because the new 'face' doesn't match the pancreas cells to spark the molecular mimicry events.

L: What if the mother cannot produce enough breast milk or due to some medical reasons during the first six months of the baby?

B: A better alternative in this case would be for the child to thrive on a surrogate mother's breast milk or breast milk from a mother's milk donor program.

L: Then for whom is it ideal to be drinking cow's milk where the chances of autoimmune fire is unlikely?

B: Baby calves of the mother cows. That's whom the cow's milk is meant for as a natural fit.

L: Okay, I think I am getting the concepts of molecular mimicry, misidentified facial match, unchecked immune fire and how gut microbiome and diet connects all these dots. How does it work for the issue I am dealing with? I have so many questions because I was just informed that my recent third episode of urinary infection had placed me into the risk category of getting a specific type of arthritis called rheumatoid arthritis[365, 366]. Both my hands are painful and stiff in the morning when I wake up.

B: Yes, your urinary infections were due to a particular type of gut bacteria called Proteus[367].

L: That's what got me all intrigued. I was told that I have to reset my gut bacteria to have more of the friendly ones or else the Proteus urinary infection will keep coming back and eventually damage my joints. I need someone to connect the dots. You said molecular mimicry plays a role in autoimmune diseases. Where does that apply to my story?

B: I think you are in the right place to connect all those dots. The first part is the connection between gut bacteria and urinary infection. That's the easy one to figure out. Anatomically for you, the end of the gut and the beginning of the urinary pathway are in close proximity, so the gut bacteria find ways to gain entry into the urethral canal to cause urinary tract infection.

The more intriguing part is why such Proteus urinary infection triggers our own immunity to attack our own joint tissues to cause auto-immune rheumatoid arthritis.

Molecular mimicry comes into play here again[368].

L: Wait, so which molecule spooks the immune system?

B: You are catching on well. The Proteus bacterium's appearance spooks the immune system, and its face gets flagged all over our immune system with bright red alert.

L: And, another tissue of my own body resembles the Proteus face? A 'friendly fire'?

B: Correct. The section of our body that takes the hit is a part of the joint which is cocooned by a gel-like connective tissue called 'synovium.' Unfortunately, the immune system sees this part of the joint and sees the same 'face' of the Proteus bacterium and releases the anti-Proteus antibodies to start the offensive[369, 370]. These antibodies are of two types and they both seem to have a connection to how healthy your gut bacterial balance is. One is anti-citrullinated antibodies[371], and the other is anti-carbamylated antibodies[372]. The latter are the same antibodies that appear to play a role in a similar joint illness ('arthritis') related to the skin problem called Psoriasis.

L: You said that these attacks go unchecked?

B: Correct. Again, the reason for the regulatory control of excessive force used by the immune system fire relates to not having adequate friendly bacteria in the gut. The lining of the gut tube has a five-layered defense barrier called the 'intestinal mucosal barrier,' where one of the layers is made of immune cells. With an imbalance of not having enough friendly bacteria, the barrier is breached, and the immune system comes into contact with unwelcome guests such as Proteus. At the same time, the regulatory control immune cells ('Tregs') that keep a check on the excessive fire don't work well without enough friendly bacteria. The result is unchecked, excessive fire on our own synovium and joint tissues, a fire similar to what was feared in Vulcan.

L: This is worrying me about my joints. I don't want this to go on to become full-blown rheumatoid arthritis in me. I may lose my job if I can't even pour coffee at the café.

B: I can tell you that this started only recently, so you may have an opportunity to take control of it.

L: Hope so, but how?

B: Well, we need to focus on two steps. One is to reduce further contact of Proteus with the immune system. In other words, ensure that there is no more urinary tract infection by Proteus. Since this Proteus is traveling from the gut to the urethra, the best place to work on this is to fix the gut's bacterial balance by ensuring enough fiber in the diet. Making sure there are enough leafy greens and beans in daily meals is known to provide the fiber that is essential for the friendly bacteria to outnumber unwelcome guests such as Proteus.

L: How long does it take after I change my meals to impact the Proteus?

B: Generally, six weeks to three months. It has been shown that switching to a plant-based diet not only reduces the footprint of Proteus in the blood circulation but also reduces the disease activity of rheumatoid arthritis[373, 374, 375, 376]. It appears that scientists are still deciding on whether there is enough evidence to recommend plant-based diets as part of treatment for autoimmune diseases. From my perspective, as the human body, I am noticing that arteries are clogging faster prematurely with early arrival of heart attacks in the setting of autoimmune diseases.[377, 378] So why delay switching to plant-based diet that can only help slow the progression and even reverse the blocking of arteries[379]?

L: Hmmm, food for thought! By the way, what is the second step?

B: This involves making sure the regulatory control over the excessive fire of the immune system works well to rein in any overreaction to the identity of mimicking molecules in the joint tissue. This involves the regulatory 'T' immune cells ("Tregs"),[380] which are in turn governed by the presence of friendly bacteria in the gut. So, essentially, both the steps involving rheumatoid arthritis can be taken care of by eating more plant-fiber in your meals[381, 382].

L: Is that why vegan or whole-food plant-based diets appear to work better for rheumatoid arthritis?

B: Correct. Also, animal foods and processed plant-foods lack dietary fiber, so every gram of such 'empty calories' replaced with unprocessed, whole plant-food only adds to the benefit of the gut bacterial balance.

L: Makes sense. I am glad I got to know about this during the early stages of this process. My friend's sister got diagnosed with multiple sclerosis at the young age of 34. How does this discussion fit with her situation?

B: Scientists who rely on large-scale research are waiting to validate what appears to be early indications from various observations showing that low-fat and higher plant-food consumption could help multiple sclerosis symptom[383]s.

L: Tell me more about the available early signals.

B: There appears to be some research showing improvement of some of the symptoms of multiple sclerosis when controlling the amount of dietary fat and when increasing more whole food plant-based meals.

L: I am interested in trying to change my diet. I just don't know if I have the willpower to maintain that.

B: Well, there are variations in perception of willpower. Some say that willpower may be finite for a given day[384, 385]. Some who cope with other aspects of their life well, like using assertive communication to express their situation or need, don't have to dip into this daily will-power budget to deal with the stress from a given situation.

L: What do you mean by this?

B: Let me explain it using an example. Let's imagine a single mother of two children working to make ends meet in her household. In the morning, there are days when her children are throwing tantrums when getting ready to go to school (more precisely, when not getting ready to go to school). Their behavior adds stress for her, but she remains calm and coaxes them to get ready with a mix of smiles and firm yet loving talk. She uses some of her willpower "budget" to hold back her reaction in that moment. Next, she goes to work and deals with clients who are demeaning and demanding or dealing with coworkers or her boss who is giving her a hard time. The work team hasn't done a great job in creating a culture of psychological safety, so she is afraid to speak up. So, instead, she puts up with it and maintains her composure and, like any good team player would in her customer service job. In doing so, she has taken more out of her daily willpower budget. She drives back home, rushing first to the daycare to pick up the kids. One is crying because he had a fight with another kid. She is there 100% for this crying kid to console him and cheer him up. As she is consoling her kids while driving, a gray car pulls suddenly in front of her from the right lane. The other driver was either under the influence of texting or another addictive substance. She wanted to honk, bring down the window and yell. She knew the kids were watching from the back seat and would learn from her behavior. With difficulty and a bigger drawing from the remaining willpower budget, she remains calm and carries on driving and talking to her kids in a smooth voice.

By the end of the day, when she returns home and finds a piece of cake or a slice of cheesecake on her kitchen table, what do you think she is going to do? She has nothing left in the will-power budget to draw from. Of course, she ends up eating a slice of cheesecake. Or two. And you are right. Of course, she can end up beating herself up for being 'weak' and for not having 'will-power like others do' which resulted in her giving into her unhealthy food choices.

One way to deal with this is by not dipping into the willpower budget pot too often in a twenty-four-hour period by learning to navigate sticky situations using assertive communication to state your need or explain your situation and ask for assistance, or by learning to say 'no.'

Also, learning to cope with stress helps with positive reframing of situations[386].

While building any and all of those skill sets, in the interim, what can also help is to re-arrange your living environment so that healthy choices such as a bowl of fruit are ready and accessible rather than cake or cheese. Don't stock your kitchen with unhealthy stuff. If you have to have an occasional treat, "hide" them. If it isn't readily reachable, even if you know where you "hid" it, you are less likely to bother with digging it out of your pantry. Bottom line: our environment and access to healthy food (in the kitchen, workplace, and neighborhoods) is a way to navigate around the need to draw from our willpower to avoid unhealthy food choices. A good reminder to stop beating yourself up ("I am weak") and start to be kind to yourself as you explore healthy choices and have that occasional slip.

L: Good reminder. I plan to start adding more unprocessed, fiber-rich, plant-based meals. It feels daunting to think about it!

B: Changing behavior is a marathon of baby steps built on with consistent practice. Remember you went white-water rafting once.

L: Yes, loved it.

B: You (we) were all padded up with the life vest. You were trying to remember the safety instructions that were given to our group as we got into the raft. That was the first rafting experience. The noise of the river was surprisingly loud compared to the quiet background scene of beautiful trees along the riverbed. Colorado River was beautiful. The water ripples gained speed despite the unsuccessful efforts by the crooked rows of rocks to stop the flow of the river. What struck us was the incredible force with which the water was moving through the rocks. It was unstoppable. It was shocking to realize the fact that this powerful force started out as a quiet trickle of spring water that was consistently flowing even though in a small volume that continued to build up to become this thundering, unstoppable force of nature. Perseverance and consistency, even with small steps, pays off. We can take a lesson from watching a river to understand that changing behavior to make healthier choices in life is about starting with small steps and maintaining that consistently to build momentum. Before we know it, the baby steps become an ultra-marathon.

Awareness, emotional memories of food, intuition, and cultural grooming play a role in our ability to make changes. Setting up the right food environment can set you up for success.

Set up and food contents of the kitchen, the design of the road, the location of grocery stores, the layout of the city regarding walkways and public transportation – all these factors influence us toward healthier behavior. If we had more farmers' markets selling fresh vegetables, we would buy them more. On the flip side, if we have more convenient stores readily accessible in front of us selling junk food and sugary drinks, we will be readily buying them instead. If our kitchen is stocked with fruit and vegetables, we are more likely to eat them. Let's now summarize what we discussed:

1. Both too little and too much immunity can harm us.
2. Too much immunity coupled with wrongly identifying self-organ as intruder leads to 'friendly fire' autoimmune attacks.
3. T-regulatory cells ('T-regs') give the command "hold the fire" so that our immune system doesn't overreact.
4. Not eating enough dietary fiber-rich foods starves our friendly bacteria and fails to stimulate production of T- regulatory cells to hold back unnecessary immune fire.
5. Dairy protein and its resemblance to insulin-producing pancreatic cells ('molecular mimicry') has been linked with diabetes that happens in children (Type 1 Diabetes).
6. Wholefood, plant-based meals treat rheumatoid arthritis.
7. Low-fat diets and increasing fiber-rich plant foods decrease symptoms of multiple sclerosis.

CHAPTER EIGHT
WORKING FRAME: JOINTS, BONES, AND MUSCLES

> Seven-word synopsis
> ***Plants strengthen bones, muscles and comfort joints***

' Hermes omnia solus et ter unus. ' [387] ('Hermes is all in one and three times great')

– Poet Marcus Valerius Martialis (1st century AD) about the Gladiator Hermes

Sarah is 65 years old. Sharp as a tack. And funny. Her mind is as active and busy as her schedule. She is a retired bookkeeper who worked for 30 years in an accounting firm. These days, she keeps busy with her volunteer work and family commitments. She is a member of her faith community's volunteer team and helps with assisting the unhoused in her neighborhood through her volunteering efforts. She is also on two committees in her community. She can contribute a lot by running the committees but can't run or even walk fast. Sadly, she can't even open a jar of pickles. Arthritis has invaded most of her joints – both the big joints in her hips and knees and the small joints next to the fingernails in her hands. Her back gives out now and then as well due to weakening of muscles around an arthritic spine. I have felt the deterioration of the joints slowly and have been waiting for this conversation for many years. What she needs is a hopeful conversation to help understand why she is riddled with arthritis and how she may be able to slow down the disease so that it doesn't slow her down to a full stop, stuck to a wheelchair. She has never been in a meditation session. She gets ready for her first meditation session.

S: Hello, it feels like I am talking to myself.

B: Yes, well, it is me, your body. During this meditation session, it is temporary, while you are in between an alert and subconscious state.

S: Glad I could sit on the reclining chair for this session. The hips and back are not easy on me. So are my knees and hands. It is a frustrating issue.

B: I know those joints are painful. I feel it every day with you.

S: Wish I could get rid of the pain. First thing in the morning when I wake up is the worst time for the joint pain. There is much I want to do in my life, and these joint issues are coming in the way of it.

B: It is true. Well, there are a few things in play in preventing further damage and/or slowing down osteoarthritis in joints - such as regular movement, keeping up with the strengthening of muscles that support the joints, and most importantly, avoiding long-term inflammation which has a lot to do with not paying attention to the food that nurtures the gut bacteria. The pain in joints such as hips and knees is made worse by making the joints carry too much load from excess body weight every minute of standing.

S: Well, what can be done at this stage of the game?

B: We can't get the joints back to their original shape. However, we can do some things to slow down the progression of the deterioration and the pain from inflammation.

S: I am all ears.

B: One thing that could help your joints and reduce your risk for cancer, heart attacks, and dementia is paying closer attention to what is on the food plate and what isn't. It can help the gut bacteria get reset to have more of the healthy bacteria and thus help with long-term inflammation[388, 389, 390, 391]. Inflammatory pain in joints is at its worst when you start to move after rest, like getting up in the morning when you wake up, as in your case.

S: Tell me more about it. I did read about inflammation. It sounded like a reaction of the body when it is hurt. Right?

B: You are correct. The injury can be from infections or trauma. It can also come from the meal plate.

S: Like when a plate falls on your foot?

B: Good one. No, I am talking about the food on the plate. But I am glad you have retained that sense of humor.

S: You got that right. But the humor only goes so far in keeping my spirit up because I can feel my body is broken. So, what about the meal plate? Go ahead and spill the beans!

B: That's a good place to start explaining this. First let me spill the arachidonic acid.

S: Whatever that acid is, don't spill it on me!

B: I've got you covered. The arachidonic acid is not the kind that can burn the skin. However, when plentiful in the body, it can provide raw material to be converted into molecules that can cause serious damage through inflammation to many organs including joints. Arachidonic acid in the tiny cells in all the organs in our body gets broken down by the cell's biological catalysts (called enzymes) that convert this molecule to harmful downstream versions. These new molecules produced from arachidonic acid's raw material have fancy scientific names, such as Prostaglandins and Leukotrienes[392]. The names are not the point. The key thing for you to know is that these newly produced molecules with their fancy names can seriously damage the cartilage in the joints by increasing inflammation in our cells. And if you are wondering what cartilage is, the gelatin-like substance lines the surface of the end of the two bones that meet together to form the joint. As long as the cartilage is healthy, we won't get arthritis. Production of these inflammatory molecules affecting the cartilage requires two things: enough raw material (arachidonic acid) and biological catalysts that go unchecked in converting the raw material to the inflammatory molecules. Logic would say that the process can be interrupted by doing two things: 1. cutting back on the supply of excessive[393] arachidonic acid coming into the body (through changes in meals) and 2. Keeping a check on the biological catalysts through medications that block the production process. Science calls option #2 non-steroidal anti-inflammatory medications taken to reduce inflammation in arthritis (for example, ibuprofen). There has been enough money put into studying the #2 process but not enough investment to study the effects of food on arthritis.

S: All of this mess originating from that acid?

B: Yes, the arachidonic acid. The one you didn't want to have spilled on you, but you eat daily.

S: What do you mean? Where is this acid in my diet?

B: Chicken, eggs, beef, pork, and lamb.[394]

S: What if I buy cage-free eggs and free-range chickens that Sally, my neighbor, always talks about?

B: Arachidonic acid is present in animal flesh regardless of situations where the chickens were extremely stressed out living in a cage or cage-free.

S: What if I cut back my eggs at breakfast?

B: That could reduce the daily dose of arachidonic acid getting into the cells.

S: That will also reduce my options for breakfast! What do I replace it with?

B: How about a tofu scramble?

S: No, thank you. It doesn't sound tasty to me.

B: Well, it may surprise you. How about trying out the Southwestern Tofu Scramble and Oil-free Crispy Hash Browns for this weekend? Or you could try fruit with high-protein grains and nuts for breakfast.

S: I don't know. I am still skeptical about the taste of the tofu scramble, but I will give it one shot! So, let me make sure I got the logic correct here. Arachidonic acid partly comes into our bodies through our food. It supplies the raw material inside the cells to be converted to molecules that facilitate inflammation – potentially even in the joints. As in my osteoarthritis. Would the opposite be true?

B: What do you mean by that?

S: Reducing the load of arachidonic acid getting into the body may lessen the osteoarthritis.

B: It is the logical conclusion we can make. Has science focused on studying this theory? It is starting to[395].

That is one aspect of the solution. The good news is that there are other areas where you can make a difference to slow down the arthritis in the joints. Have you heard of endotoxins?

S: The word toxins is telling me something anyway.

B: You are correct. The "endo" in that word means inside. That is something that works in the inner workings of the body. Endotoxin is more recently called 'Lipo-polysaccharides' because they are made of crumbled 'skin' of bacteria in the gut[396]. Lipopolysaccharides (LPS), on release, can increase inflammation in the joint tissues such as cartilage as well as tissues of other organs. LPS can take a manageable situation such as abscess or infection into becoming life-threatening whole-body infection ('sepsis') in the right setting where the human body is weak and under duress. A classic example is the millions of war wounds that turned into fatal infections in ancient armies,[397] essentially changing history by tipping the victory to the army with fewer deaths from wound infection. LPS, despite determining geo-political history through outcome of wars remained under the radar until the 'golden age of microbiology[398], the later part of 19th century. In 1876, Robert Koch, a German microbiologist discovered bacteria. It will take another eighteen years of collaboration between Koch and another German physician Richard Pfeiffer of Berlin to discover endotoxin in 1894[399, 400].

Protecting the cartilage is key because the fundamental problem with arthritis is the damage to the cartilage and the associated inflammation. One of the things that affect the cartilage is the endotoxin aka LPS[401].

S: What triggers the releases of these endotoxins?

B: High-fat diets which are popular in "low-carbohydrate diets". The other reason is not having enough dietary fiber[402]. Diets high in saturated fat[403, 404] and low in fiber contribute to high blood levels of these endotoxins through several mechanisms, including changes in the gut bacterial population[405].

S: Okay, I will work on reducing the arachidonic acid and endotoxins in my meals. I will work on reducing the butter during breakfast time. Anything else?

B: Wow, I am impressed by how much motivation the joint pains can bring for someone to change their meal style. One last thing we need to talk about is the impact of body fat.

S: I know. I have a big belly. That is no secret.

B: The good news is that diet changes to increase dietary fiber with more of wholefood plant-based meals will start to reduce the excess fat in its most troublesome area - deep in the abdomen. A location called visceral fat. It is the fat hugging the intestines, deeper than the fat just beneath the skin over the abdomen.

S: So, there is a second layer of fat underneath the skin of the abdomen.

B: Correct. And that visceral fat is like a factory for inflammation that keeps churning inflammatory molecules into the body's systems. Having excess visceral fat increases arthritis. When visceral fat shrinks, it reduces inflammation in the body.[406]

S: It appears that the same diet changes will reduce the inflammation from LPS, visceral fat, and reduce excess arachidonic acid.

B: Correct. One approach to address several strategies of reducing inflammation of osteoarthritis. The excess body weight also places an extraordinary physical burden (load) on joints, especially knees, hips, and backbones. This makes the arthritis worse in weight-bearing joints such as knee joints. There are sensors in the joints and cartilage that are sensitive to physical (mechanical) pressure. These sensors are called 'mechano-sensitive receptors.[407]' In the knees, they sense the excess weight carried by the overweight person and trigger a change in cells' genetic command to produce more inflammation in the cartilage in the joints.

S: Does this mean that making changes to my diet could not only reduce the load of arachidonic acid and supply more fiber for the gut bacteria to prevent endotoxins but also may help lose body weight and its effect on weight-bearing joints such as knees?

B: Correct. Changing your meals can work through many mechanisms to limit inflammation and arthritis. For instance, for every additional pound of body weight, the physical load on the knees turns out to be four pounds[408]. So, if you think about it, if someone has an excess of 10 pounds, their knees feel an excess of 40 pounds whenever they are standing or walking. For the knees, it is like carrying an extra 40 pounds of bags when you are walking.

On the flip side, anytime someone sheds excess body weight, the benefit on the knee quadruples. If one sheds 5 pounds, they take 20 pounds off their knees. Imagine if someone loses 30 pounds, taking 120 pounds of load off their knees. This would be like someone was carrying 120 lbs of bags every minute of standing or walking in life and now decided to drop the bags and walk free. That's how the knees feel with the weight loss.

S: That is a great deal for the knees! Lose one pound and take four off the knees.

B: So, based on this off-loading for the joints that take the pressure off the weight-bearing joints, every meal choice is an unconscious or conscious decision to drive convenience for the knee and hip joints: more dietary fiber, less sugar and fats, and more convenience for the knees and hips.

Additionally, if this weight loss involves shrinking the visceral fat, the inflammation in the body decreases as well, thus helping the arthritic knees.

S: It is too bad that things started to get worse in the past four years with weight gain and joint pain when I started to have more financial comfort at the end of my working career. Right when I wanted to have more time for myself to enjoy life, I find myself not able to physically do many things due to the state of my health.

B: It is common that certain long-term illnesses arrive with changing lifestyle driven by new access to low-nutrient, high-calories food and snacks after growing up with not enough resources.

S: Kind of a release phenomenon?

B: Correct. It is not a new concept. It dates back to 10th and 11th century sculptures that tell the story of Kubera[409], the god of wealth according to ancient Hindu scriptures from India. He is also considered the god-king of nature-spirits (called Yakshas) who are caretakers of the natural resources under the earth, as in the roots of trees. Kubera is a symbol of wealth. Sculptures show how he is adorned with jewelry. Interestingly, he is always depicted in sculptures dating back to 2000 B.C. as obese. Yes, even then, obesity was associated with increased wealth. Beyond Hindu religion, Kubera's sculptures appeared in other religions that began in India, such as Buddhism and Jainism. Regardless of which religion Kubera is depicted in, he is portrayed as obese. Now, scientific research has confirmed the strong correlation between increasing wealth in a community and an increase in obesity and related chronic diseases, regardless of which country or culture. When wealth increases, it has been shown to increase the obesity rate in that country or culture. Part of the reason is the 'double burden of malnutrition.' This involves the release phenomenon you correctly identified, where someone grows up in poverty without adequate access to food and overcompensates when wealth and access to food increases. It is a deep-seated biological drive that tries to quickly pack as much energy in fats as possible for a potential future famine. Another paradox is what is called the 'food insecurity-obesity paradox.[410]' This is driven by the built environment and food system that makes cheap calories available without adequate nutrition. A person who is currently in poverty and is unable to have food on the table on a daily basis may resort to these cheaply available high-calorie, low-nutrient fast-food meals. This leads to obesity in the setting of poverty and inadequate nutrition[411].

S: I always wondered about that. I get the paradox now.

B: The type of ingredients in these meals also lack the nourishment that the gut bacteria need, thus altering the gut-bacterial balance. The resulting imbalance in the gut bacteria perpetuates the problem of obesity in the setting of poor nutrition.

Not able to put food on the table or *nutrient-rich* food on the table with access only to cheap, high-calorie, low-nutrient fast food - both have the same effect on excess weight gain. Social determinants of health such as 'food swamp' neighborhoods[412] filled with stores that sell cheap, high-calorie food with no physical access to nutritious food and discrimination-driven systemic lack of opportunities for education and livelihood that result in poverty are some of the factors that drive food 'choices' (or the lack of). Such communities have 'food deserts' and are inherently 'nutrient deserts.'

Resulting in excess calories, poor nutrition leading to poor gut bacterial balance, and consequently weight gain - all raise the burden on knees. The result is osteoarthritis arriving sooner in these individuals.

S: Okay, let me see if I can summarize what you said.

1. Abnormal mechanical loading on the weight-bearing joints can lead to inflammation and osteoarthritis - as in excess weight gain or repetitive sports injuries. This is mediated by the "pressure sensors" in the cartilage, which has another fancy name.

2. Arachidonic acid - the raw material that gets into our body through food, resulting in a chain of events leading to inflammation - which is blocked by medications such as ibuprofen, and let me see....

3. LPS or 'Endotoxins' are released from our gut lining due to starvation of friendly bacteria that can no longer prevent a breakdown of the gut lining.

4. Visceral fat releases inflammation and shrinking it with high fiber plant foods helps reduce inflammation overall.

5. Living situations, such as not having access to nutritious calories in food or past experiences of poverty turned later into affluence, can determine food choices as in the 'food insecurity-weight gain paradox.'

B: You were paying attention.

S: What if I follow your advice and start eating to limit arthritis but miss the nutrients I need to keep my bones strong? Looks like I will be cutting back on most of the proteins I am used to and start eating more dietary fiber-rich foods. My doctor told me that I have osteoporosis. The bones started to show this soon after I hit menopause.

B: What do you imagine your new meals to be? Give me an example.

S: Protein that has dietary fiber and vegetables that the gut bacteria like so that they can keep guarding the gut lining to prevent endotoxins?

B: Perhaps protein, as in beans or chickpeas and leafy greens, as part of the meals?

S: We are a good team figuring these things out. I just need to pay more attention to your messages!

B: Good choice. That combination is also great for your bone health.

S: You mean chickpeas and green salad? There is no milk or dairy in it. How can that be good for bone health without dairy?

B: Well, the understanding of nutrition for bone health has changed considerably in the past two decades.

S: Really, are you serious? Why is everything changing about what we know about food? Is there anything that has not changed regarding our health and food?

B: Well, don't worry. Leafy greens and vegetables are still the best thing on the plate.

S: At least something is unchanged!

B: The change in view of bone health is a big one. In the early days, 30-40 years ago, the advice from government health departments used to be that drinking milk and eating dairy was the only way and the best way to get strong bones. The science of understanding bone health has changed over the years. Now, we know that bone health does not rely solely on calcium.

S: Similar to "most valuable player' used in sports?

B: Correct. In the bone health and nutrients game, no single most valuable player or "player of the match." In science, we have realized that nutrients other than calcium are equally important[413, 414] such as potassium, magnesium[415], Vitamin K, and Vitamin D are all important for bone health. Among these nutrients, Vitamin D is best obtained naturally from sunlight. Depending upon the geographical location and the amount of melanin pigment on one's skin, the amount of sunlight exposure needed to get enough Vitamin D naturally can vary. Concerning the other nutrients important for bone health such as potassium, Vitamin K[416], and Magnesium,[417] eating beans and dark green leafy vegetables regularly is a better solution than milk or dairy because the wholesome plant foods also bring in dietary fiber that is absent in milk and dairy.

S: That is news for me. I never thought that beans and greens would strengthen my bone health.

B: Other important nutrients for bone health are present in greens and beans but absent in milk and dairy.

S: Other than the list that you just told me?

B: Protein that comes with dietary fiber: it is a double-edged sword when it comes to bone health. Too much protein can hurt, as would too little.

S: Hmm, tell me more about it.

B: You see, protein has a bone-building effect. Eating protein stimulates something called Insulin-like Growth Factor-1. We will call it IGF-1. This substance stimulates something called Osteocalcin, which promotes bone growth and increases the density of the bones. This is all nice. But if someone consumes too much of this protein, especially animal protein, it brings in too much sulfur into the mix, creating an acidic environment[418]. Bone doesn't like an acidic environment in the body because this acidity will leach calcium off the bones to neutralize the acid[419, 420]. So, eating too much animal protein can be detrimental to the bones. These folks could benefit from scaling back on the excess animal protein and adding more beans, vegetables and fruit[421]. Some researchers believe that the positive and negative effect of high protein in diet may cancel out each other when they note "opposing anabolic (uptake of calcium by the gut, impact on IGF-1) and catabolic actions of dietary protein (increase of acidic load of diet) may cancel each other out to some extent."[422]

Remember, I said double-edged sword. Yes, too little protein in meals can also hurt the bones. If someone is eating not enough calories, they can run into protein deficiency. In these folks the lack of adequate protein leads to a lack of IGF-1 stimulation of the bones. This can lead to not having enough density built for the bones. So, for an omnivore eating too much animal protein, the best thing is to eliminate or drastically cut down on animal protein and increase the intake of fruits and vegetables. On the other hand, for a vegan who doesn't eat enough calories, they need to make sure they eat adequate calories and protein in order to maintain bone health. Such a person choosing mostly or exclusively plant-derived food, making sure enough calories are consumed from a variety of plant-food sources will ensure that adequate protein is provided.

S: Very interesting! What is the deal with eating more leafy greens, vegetables, and fruit for bone health?

B: Yes. Something vital for bone health is abundant in fruit and vegetables - including leafy greens: The anti-oxidants.

S: Wait a minute. Antioxidants that I learned to be useful to prevent cancer? Are you sure you are not mixing up bone health with cancer? I know I didn't sleep well last night. Maybe, that is messing up your thinking?

B: That is funny. No, I am not mixing up my thoughts here. Yes, the same antioxidants that help prevent cancer and heart attacks also help maintain good bone health. Anti-oxidants have everything to do with why women get osteoporosis during menopause.[423, 424]

S: Isn't menopausal osteoporosis due to a lack of estrogen in the women's body? I thought it was related to hormone levels.

B: Yes and no. Yes, it is related to estrogen hormone levels. When the woman reaches menopausal age, the ovaries don't produce enough estrogen, and hence, the blood level of this hormone drops. However, this results in osteoporosis among some women because they do not have enough antioxidants in their bodies.

S: What does the timing of estrogen level dropping during menopause have to do with a lack of antioxidants?

B: They are the same. Recent discoveries have shown that estrogens have antioxidant capacity and protect bone health[425]. Everyday routine inside our bone cells builds up certain amounts of toxins called oxidants. These are also known as free radicals. These toxic molecules accumulate more when the body (that is me) is exposed to polluting chemicals and stress (physical and emotional)[426, 427]. As long as the woman has an adequate level of estrogen produced in the body, the estrogen's antioxidant capacity can prevent the oxidants from damaging and weakening the bones. However, when menopause hits, the levels drop and speed up the development of osteoporosis if the woman is not eating enough colorful fruits and vegetables to supply anti-oxidants. The speed of osteoporosis unfolding in their bodies depends upon how deficient they are in antioxidant capacity in their blood.

S: That sounds convenient. Looks like the same antioxidant foods that help with bone health are also the ones that help with muscle recovery after exercise.

B: Yes, muscles and bones are happy when they feed me with antioxidant-rich food. Those rich colors of leafy greens, beets, sweet potato, peppers, tomatoes, fruit, and all the other yummy stuff! These foods also supply other nutrients important for bone strength, such as magnesium and potassium.

S: Okay, and isn't exercise also good for the bones?

B: Yes, as they say, use it or lose it. The more active we are every day, the better for me. Strength training or activities that pose a load on the bones are especially important for the bones to maintain their strength[428].

S: Can you explain what you mean by the load on the bone?

B: It is about how hard the bone works during movement. If someone lifts their arm with nothing in their hands, that is not putting much load on the arm bone except for the weight of the arm itself. On the other hand, if the same person is lifting something heavy using their hands, their bone is working hard against the weight and gravity to lift it up. The hard work the bone is doing is due to the load on the bone. That is what I mean. There are some more details to this. It also matters as to how many directions the load is coming from[429]. Whether it is just in one direction, as in walking, running, or bicycling, or whether the load is occurring in multiple directions, as with someone who is playing volleyball, who, maybe unknowingly, is placing the load on their leg bones and spine from different directions due to the way the game itself makes them turn, twist, jump and land- as they play the sport.

S: Jumping, too!

B: Yes, I love when people jump. My bony parts get a little shock, a good shock that helps my bone system to maintain its strength - much like the multi-directional load on the bones. Jump rope is a typical example. When I am made to jump rope, I feel the good effect on my bones. Technically, it is called "ground reaction force[430, 431]". One of the prescriptions for young people is to jump rope 30-100 jumps at least three times a week to maintain good bone strength. The ancient civilizations in India seem to have figured this out thousands of years ago.

S: Really? How?

B: The classical dance from Tamil Nadu, India, is called Barathanaatiyam[432]. The dance involves intricate footwork, rhythms, and expressions woven together in the choreography to tell stories through dance movements. It is an ancient art practiced for over two thousand years. One of the frequent and common moves in this dance is where the dancer jumps and lands on her/his feet. Interestingly enough, this dance is practiced mostly by women who stand to benefit from the "ground reaction force" of the jumps involved in this traditional dance.

S: 'Jump to benefit' would be more accurate than "stand to benefit"!

B: Good one! And there are many other dance traditions globally that also involve jumping, honestly too many to list but some examples include Ballet, Adumu dance of Africa, Capoeira from Brazil, the Irish Jig and so on. Moreover, any dance has the ability to place mechanical load on the bones from many directions.

S: Funny! What about other sports for bone health?

B: Well, any sports that will make someone move in all directions with or without jumping can help: tennis, squash, cross-country skiing. Though not studied, I feel that dancing and yoga, which can also load the bones from different directions, are likely to help the same way volleyball can. Future research may show that one can dance one's way into avoiding osteoporosis.

S: So, for bone health, how important is physical activity and load on bone compared to nutrition?

B: More than 50 % of the contribution to good bone health comes from physical activity, especially what someone does before they reach 30[433]. Nutrition is almost equally important. Adequate calcium, protein, potassium, magnesium, Vitamin K, and Vitamin D intake is key in nutrition.

S: Wait. I am older than 30. Does that mean it is too late for my bones to get stronger?

B: Well, it is not hopeless. You still have twenty to thirty percentage room to work with to improve your bone health after age 30. Nearly seventy percentage of the adult's bone density is determined by age 30.

S: So, antioxidant-rich colorful fruits and vegetables, dark greens and beans, and a jump rope. Is that the way to roll?

B: Yes, if someone can't safely do jump rope or play one of these sports, then simple weight training for the big muscles of hips, arms, back, and abdomen will be an alternative.

S: So what would you like to be fed before and after I work out?

B: Simple. Before the workout, fruit, vegetables, whole grains (rice, pasta, bread), with some nuts[434]. Healthy starch from the fruit, vegetables, or whole grains and good fats from the nuts or nut butter. That will fuel the muscles well when making them work hard. After working out, a colorful salad or cooked vegetable dish with various colorful vegetables for anti-oxidant source and lentils or beans and nuts/seeds or quinoa for amino acids to rebuild the muscles broken down during the workout.

S: Good to know the difference between pre-and post-workout nutritional needs for the body. Let me make sure I can recall and summarize what I heard you say about bone health. Lack of antioxidants is at the root of osteoporosis, resulting in low bone mass and weak bones. Colorful vegetables, leafy greens, and fruits boost antioxidants in meals. Adequate calories and protein are key, and meeting the protein needs through beans and legumes can supply the dietary fiber for healthy gut bacteria to keep inflammation of joints in check and to supply the protein needed and ensure the supply of other elements important for bone health, such as magnesium and potassium. What about Vitamin D that I read about?

S: The geographical location of where one lives will determine how much Vitamin D that person will get from the sun - the most powerful stimulus for Vitamin D production under our skin. Those who live in countries and regions away from the Equator, north or south of the 37th parallel latitude line[435], will need to make sure the food is fortified with Vitamin D or take a supplement that has 1000 international units of Vitamin D. The regions in the middle of the Earth's globe, hugging the Equator that is between the north 37th parallel latitude and south 37th parallel latitude, provide plenty of sunshine all year round to make daily Vitamin D. For simplicity, let's call this the 'Vitamin D belt' that goes around the globe.

S: Sun exposure also causes skin damage and skin cancer for those who don't have enough melanin pigment in their skin.

B: Correct. You can have Vitamin D from the sun and avoid skin damage from the sun. The good news is that you don't need to be out in the sun all day to get enough Vitamin D. Just 10 to 15 minutes of exposure to arms and legs a few times a week is enough to produce enough Vitamin D.[436] In countries outside the 'Vitamin D belt,' this is possible in the summer months. During the rest of the year, people here must rely on fortified food sources or Vitamin D supplements.

S: Got it. To make sure, I will pick up a Vitamin D supplement for the non-summer months. Does that cover all that I need to know about my bone health?

B: It covers the basics of nutrients and bone health. Let's not forget the neighbors of the bones.

S: Who?

B: Muscles. They are part of the team that makes up your framework, bone, and joints. Working together, this team helps you to move and do all your activities. Muscle mass and strength is as important as bone mass and strength in the context of fractures, falls, and quality of life. Have you heard of something called Sarcopenia?

S: No. Tell me about it.

B: Loss of muscle bulk and function is called sarcopenia[437]. It is a common condition among elders regardless of whether they live in Salem in India, England, or the United States. It can also happen in younger people if they have conditions such as cancer, AIDS, or tuberculosis. Sarcopenia doesn't get as much attention as osteoporosis, even though it is equally important to stabilize the bone/joint framework to prevent falls and fractures.[438]

S: How does this 'Sarcopenia' show up in the body?

B: Older adults with sarcopenia experience increased risk of frailty, disability, hospitalizations, mortality, increased risk of falls, increased risk of fractures, longer length of stay in the hospital after fracture, worse results after surgery for fracture, and reduced quality of life. The most common reason for sarcopenia is poor nutrition[439, 440] and lack of physical activity[441], especially strength training for the muscles[442].

S: So, what are the nutritional aspects one needs to pay attention to for preventing sarcopenia?

B: There are five goals in the nutritional approach to prevent sarcopenia[443]:

1. Eating adequate food and enough calories
2. Avoid protein deficiency by aiming slightly higher protein intake such as 15% of daily caloric need (preferably plant-origin due to benefits to other co-existing illnesses, kidneys, colon and bowel health etc.)
3. Adequate anti-oxidant intake through colorful fruit and vegetables
4. Anti-inflammatory approach with more omega-3 fatty acids and less animal protein and high fat food, wherein the latter two can injure gut lining and trigger inflammation.
5. Alignment of approach with improving gut microbiome and overall metabolic health such as that of blood sugar, cholesterol, heart health, kidney health etc.

S: It looks like there are similarities with the dietary approach to address osteoarthritis.

B: Logic would say that good nutrition also keeps other metabolic parameters in a good range - such as LDL cholesterol, blood pressure, blood sugar, etc. Evidence also points to the correlation between sarcopenia and poor levels of these metabolic parameters[444].

B: On the flip side, people who live in blue zones or centenarian cultures avoid sarcopenia a great deal due to their good practices of healthy nutrition and active lifestyle. They also have excellent longevity due to healthy metabolic profiles[445] regarding cholesterol levels, blood sugar, and blood pressure. That is why they are putting up roofs and working in the farm fields when they are in their 90s.[446]

S: So, eating healthy and moving your joints and muscles can help reduce risk factors for heart attack, stroke, and cancers and maintain muscle bulk! That sounds like a nice package deal. But what about the protein? Can I take extra protein supplements to prevent sarcopenia?

B: Not so fast. Researchers have reviewed all the studies on the association between sarcopenia and physical activity with or without protein supplements to understand which factors worked to prevent or improve muscle loss (bulk and function). As expected, physical activity was confirmed to contribute to enhancing muscle mass. Still, the study failed to show significant improvement in muscle function and bulk in the studies that tried different vitamin and protein supplementation[447]. Why didn't these research interventions with supplements work compared to those living in blue zones or centenarian cultures? The people living in these centenarian cultures eat whole food, mostly plant food, with 95 to 100% of their protein coming from plant foods[448]. Their food is rich in micronutrients such as antioxidants, phytochemicals, and other vitamins. The protein and vitamin supplementation provided in the research settings doesn't compare with the comprehensive style of the package of naturally available whole food.

With regard to physical activity for sarcopenia, the strongest evidence of benefit is shown with strength training exercises, especially in the elderly population.

Eating the wholefood, plant-based way like the centenarians do will prevent sarcopenia and obesity.

S: Can these two co-exist?

B: The condition is called 'sarcopenic obesity.'[449] It is the worst of both worlds combined. The decline in function is much worse for elders who have a combination of obesity and sarcopenia than those having one of these two conditions. A perfect storm for falling and breaking bones[450]. A landmark research study[451] led by French researcher Yves Rolland confirmed this. Four groups of elderly women were compared. Those who had normal body weight, another group with obesity, a third group with sarcopenia alone, and the fourth group with both sarcopenia and obesity. Compared with the group with normal body weight, the obese group had 47% more impairment in function as measured by their ability to climb stairs. The sarcopenic group had 79% more impairment in climbing stairs. The group that had both sarcopenia and obesity had the worse outcome: 260% worse impairment in climbing stairs compared with the normal body weight group.

S: That sounds like double trouble for physical ability and risk of falling when one has both obesity and sarcopenia. Solution?

B: A successful twin-strategy for sarcopenic obesity is being physically active and meeting the needs of daily calories and protein by eating meals rich in micronutrients – whole food plant based meals for the most part. This is an area where clear and documented evidence is lacking about the combination of diet and exercise for sarcopenic obesity. More research is needed, but looking at successful populations such as centenarian cultures is a good place to start understanding solutions. It is important to make sure the nutrient needs are met while trying to address obesity in a patient with sarcopenia. Achieving weight loss in this population should be approached carefully to ensure that the strategies don't worsen sarcopenia while attempting to reduce obesity.

S: The observations from the centenarian cultures sound good, but I am still skeptical. Has any other evidence shown that eating plant foods helps bones, joints, and muscles? It is hard for me get past the idea that is ingrained in me that we need meat and dairy to build muscles and bones.

B: Perhaps we should look at the diet of the perfectly sculpted, agile, strong-as-an-ox warriors who roamed parts of the planet during the Roman empire: the gladiators. They were anything but frail. Their risk of fracture was related to injuries from staged blood-pumping fights in the grand spectacle stage, such as the Colosseum. Their diet was designed to render their bones with a high threshold for breaking and, if broken, to heal swiftly.

S: Gladiators! I have seen them in movies. What do we know factually about them? How can we learn about their health and diet when they have been gone for many centuries? I don't think we have their electronic health records to analyze their data.

B: By studying their bones, which keep a long-standing nutrition record[452] by revealing the composition of minerals still retained in the bone structure even centuries later.

S: Interesting! Which minerals did they study?

B: Carbon, Nitrogen, Calcium, Strontium and Sulfur. Carbon content in the bones indicate the amount of plant foods consumed by the individual. Nitrogen reflects the amount of animal protein consumed. Calcium and Strontium to assess the availability of minerals contributing to the strength of bones.

S: And what did the researchers find?

B: The composition of the bone minerals indicates that the primary diet of gladiators was made of barley, wheat, beans, and vegetables. The low nitrogen content of the bones also indicates that their meat and dairy consumption was negligible.

Wheat, barley, beans, and vegetables are rich sources of the safer, non-radioactive type of strontium that helps build up bone mass.

S: Are you saying that the gladiators, who were fighters with immense physical strength, ate primarily barley, wheat, beans, and vegetables?

B: Correct. The variety in plant meals and adequate supply of calories to meet the demands of physical training are required nutritionally to build one's body to be a gladiator.

S: That's a revelation for me. So, you don't need to eat meat and dairy to become strong?

B: Correct. Contemporary Roman texts written about gladiators corroborate with what the bone findings showed. The texts describe the above diet of gladiators as *'gladiatoriam saginam'*[453]. Most of the gladiators died young due to the fights. However, bone research shows how their diet kept them strong for training and fights. On the other extreme of the age spectrum, the centenarian cultures showed how individuals in their 90s and 100s were active with a great quality of life due to a similar diet primarily made of vegetables, whole grains, beans, and lentils.

S: That's hopeful to know that one can age healthily.

B: Aging is not about an increase in the number of birthdays. It is rather about the increase in discord in the perfectly orchestrated physiological symphony inside human cells. Let's now summarize the key points:

1. Osteoarthritis – Arachidonic acid load comes from consuming chicken, eggs, beef, pork, lamb.
2. Protecting the cartilage in joints helps prevent osteoarthritis.
3. Lipopolysaccharides (LPS) also known as 'endotoxins' destroy joint cartilage by increasing inflammation.
4. High-fat and low-dietary fiber in meals increase LPS.
5. 'Visceral fat' due to excess calories also increases inflammation.
6. Excess body weight is sensed by the joint sensors and that in turn, triggers more inflammation in the cartilage in the joints.
7. For every pound of weight gain, the knees feel 4 pounds.
8. Dietary fiber, less sugar/fat comforts and protects the joints.
9. Osteoporosis: Beans and leafy greens strengthen bones.
10. Vitamin D helps bones: from supplement or sunlight, depending upon living area.
11. Antioxidants, colorful fruit and vegetables, prevent post-menopausal bone loss.
12. Too little or too much protein – both undermine bones.
13. Sarcopenia: Inadequate dietary protein and absent strength training weakens muscles / increases risk of fall and fractures.
14. Fall risk is worse when sarcopenia coexists with obesity.
15. Gladiators' diet menu: Beans, vegetables, wheat and barley!

CHAPTER NINE
MEMORY SAVINGS FOR THE FUTURE: BRAIN HEALTH

> Seven-word synopsis
> ***Plant foods prevent and improve Alzheimer's disease***

Peter: Maybe I am just exhausted. Trying this meditation feels like I am talking to myself.

Body: Peter, correct. You are talking to me, your body.

Peter: Is this kind of where I start losing my marbles? I was afraid of memory loss catching up to me after seeing what happened to my dad.

B: No, your brain is fine. Meditation's effect on the brain is the exact opposite. Mindfulness meditation improves attention [454, 455, 456, 457, 458, 459] and memory [460, 461, 462, 463, 464, 465, 466]. This meditation took you into a trance, sometimes called a hypnotic state, and here we are, ready for a good chat. Your dad's dementia was an unfortunate turning point in your family. As his caretaker, you have a lot on your plate. You are doing a great job at it, though. By the way, great going on the extempore performance when your dad comes up with new scenarios that his mind is imagining to be reality.

P: You seem to know my story. I hope this, our little chat here, isn't one of my imaginations.

B: Trust me. You are fine. You will soon snap out of this internal conversation when the suspended mind returns to reality.

P: Oh, good. Yes, I am becoming better at playing any role I am given in this game of extempore that I find myself in often - out of necessity from dad's disease. Initially, I had no clue how to handle it. Dad will suddenly come up with the notion that there are hundreds of birds inside the room when there are none, and I would keep correcting him without knowing that there is no good that comes of correcting him[467] when dementia is driving that behavior. Another day, he may conjure up the scene where his neighbor Andy sneaks behind the bed to "steal" his watch. If it is a romantic scene, it is usually that Mom, who passed away ten years ago, is wearing a beautiful flowery dress in bright blue and white as she walks toward him with her typical laughter that sounds like a gentle clash of wind chimes on a calm, breezy evening. Of course, none of these scenes are real. They are grand imageries conjured up by broken brain cells that folded under the weight of Alzheimer's dementia.

B: Do you get tired of it?

P: Of what? The role plays?

B: Yes, it has been four years now, I believe.

P: Do I get tired of it? Sometimes. Will I quit doing it? No. Unless it is unsafe for him, I need to be there to go along with his stories. I still remember the dementia support group class that I was attending four years ago. I never thought we would be role-playing on a stage under the guidance of a drama theater director who taught us the art of extempore. Little did I know that we should not correct patients with dementia when they imagine themselves and us to be in unreal situations. People with dementia are in ever-changing scenes, and every time we correct them that there are no birds in the room, that Mom isn't here, and she's been dead for ten years – every time we do this, we chip away at their dignity and make them feel more depressed and worthless. You can see that disappointment in their eyes. So, yes, I am getting good at going along with the flow of stories.

B: What did you learn from the experience of caring for your dad, Charlie?

P: Life is a series of discoveries, which we call experiences and relationships, strung together. Life got more blessed for me when I started to learn from those discoveries, staying open to change, and making room for self-growth and self-care.

B: I am glad you are doing what you can to avoid that same fate happening to you as it did to your dad.

P: I would have waited longer until I became sixty or sixty-five to start choosing a healthier way of living, but that self-care lecture by the doctor in the caretaker support group meeting changed my life.

B: It is like investing now for future benefit. Who would have known that what we eat in our forties and fifties can be the dealmaker for dementia risk when we get to our seventies or eighties?

P: It was very interesting that it is not much different from saving for retirement funds such as 401(K).

B: Can you explain more?

P: The idea of saving for thirty or forty years down the line by putting money today in retirement funds for the future is something the majority of people do. But most people don't think that way when it comes to saving brain cells by eating better today in their middle age. I have realized that avoiding sugary food and eating vegetables, whole grains, nuts, and seeds is the 401(K) to saving your marbles for the future, which means preserving the mind[468, 469].

B: 401(K) for the brain! The evidence seems to be piling up on this notion. People with high levels of inflammation in the setting of pre-diabetes in middle age have a 66% higher risk of getting dementia when they get older[470]. And the beauty is that this inflammation can be curtailed by changing what is on your plate[471]. Likewise, what matters for the brain is maintaining a steady, normal blood sugar level by choosing healthy carbohydrates instead of sugar and processed carbohydrates. When blood sugars are high, the body produces more insulin to counter this high sugar level. The high insulin environment is not healthy for the brain cells[472, 473]. Research on the brains of patients who died with dementia shows that every change inside the brain cell that is characteristic of Alzheimer's dementia is associated with high insulin levels. When the cells of a brain afflicted with such dementia are studied under a microscope, the signature of high insulin levels is everywhere. If high blood sugar is detrimental to the brain due to high insulin levels, low blood sugar also damages the brain's memory capacity. The brain will struggle without healthy levels of blood glucose.

P: Did you say something about inflammation going hand in hand with such high insulin levels in the blood when memory cells get burned? It appears that avoiding inflammation is also key to preserving memory.

B: Yes. The main pillars of inflammation in the food are arachidonic acid, visceral fat, and endotoxins also called Lipopolysaccharides, all of which can be minimized by choosing more of a wholefood, plant-based meal pattern. 401(Ks) for the brain come in the form of fresh fruit for snacks instead of cookies, veggie burgers instead of hamburgers, omega-3 fatty acid rich flax-meal sprinkled in breakfast or salads in place of eggs, lentil sliders instead of sloppy joes, chickpea salad instead of chicken salad, and so on. What is efficient about this meal pattern is that in addition to preventing Alzheimer's dementia, it also helps treat mild stages of this dementia even after diagnosis.

P: This is groundbreaking news that there is a solution to treat Alzheimer's disease and that too using lifestyle changes.

B: New exciting research[474] just confirmed that wholefood, plant meals combined with regular relaxation, staying active, having regular social interactions improved memory in patients with mild dementia. What works for Alzheimer's disease also works for vascular dementia.

P: What is vascular dementia?

B: It is a type of dementia caused by blockage in the arterial blood flow to the brain[475]. It can happen following a noticeable event such as a stroke in the brain or it can happen gradually from blockage of many tiny arteries that supply oxygen and nutrients to the brain. Sort of like many silent mini-brain attacks that over a period of time damage enough brain tissue areas to start manifesting as memory problems.

P: How common is this vascular dementia?

B: Around thirty to forty percentage of dementia in the population is solely due to vascular dementia[476]. Among patients with Alzheimer's dementia, vascular dementia contributes to the memory problem in sixty percent of those individuals[477]. Luckily, diets high in plant nutrients [478, 479] lower the risk of vascular dementia.

P: After seeing what my dad is going through, I never want to do anything that would increase my risk for dementia. I am surprised by how tasty and fun these new foods are. Knowing that this new way of eating can reduce inflammation and avoid pre-diabetes is my best 401(K) investment. Preserving my marbles is a priceless investment.

B: Some might say, what good is it to have a big bank balance to spend when seeing imaginary things while unable to dress oneself or lose the ability to drive a vehicle safely?

P: And it is good that fruit and vegetables can help. But isn't it too late for me, since the risk is probably already there, with my dad's genetic influence on my health outcomes?

B: The horse is not entirely out of the barn. You heard that right. It doesn't matter if you have a genetic risk to get Alzheimer's dementia. You have the power to change your direction and avoid the risk. Researchers analyzed thirty years of data from the Swedish Twin Registry to study how many get dementia and their food habits[480]. It is important to note that fifty of the twin pairs studied were discordant for dementia diagnosis. In other words, even though they were identical twins, only one of the twins in these fifty pairs developed dementia after following for thirty years. Reasoning implies that factors other than genetics, such as lifestyle and diet, drove the outcome from the seed planted by the gene.

P: Interesting. What did the researchers find?

B: Researchers found that compared to the difference in intake of certain food groups between twin siblings, the difference noted in the consumption of fruits and vegetables significantly reduced the risk of developing dementia in those who didn't develop it after thirty years of observation. The risk was cut down by nearly half even after adjusting for differences in other factors (among the twins) that could contribute to such an effect, for example, age, smoking status, exercise level, body weight, total daily caloric intake, etc. This protective effect of fruit and vegetables was even more pronounced in women and those with evidence of heart disease.

P: Aren't fruit and vegetables in the carbohydrate category?

B: Yes.

P: It is so confusing for the public. Most of them avoid carbohydrates to address blood sugar or body weight problems. Here, you are saying blood sugar problems, high insulin levels, and inflammation are connected to memory problems. In the twin study, fruit and vegetable consumption reduced the risk of dementia, even in those with genetic risk. Does this mean that to protect the memory cells, one has to risk diabetes?

B: Let's unpack what you just said because some assumptions are built in there. The confusion comes from lumping all carbohydrates, such as processed flour and sugar, and healthy, wholesome fruit, vegetables, legumes, and whole grains into the same bucket. Eating healthy carbohydrates can not only help prevent diabetes but also reduce the risk of dementia—one solution for both problems.

P: Unprocessed fruit and vegetables. Got it.

B: Correct. They contain several compounds with antioxidant and anti-inflammatory properties, such as vitamins C and E, carotenoids, and polyphenols, that are non-vitamin antioxidants more potent than conventional vitamins, which are thought to protect brain cells by reducing insulin swings, wear and tear of the cells, and by quelling the fire of inflammation. Let's not forget that the dietary fiber in wholesome vegetables and some fruits is also helpful in avoiding high insulin levels.

P: How can dietary fiber that helps avoid constipation help with memory? I am intrigued!

B: The gut bacteria[481, 482, 483]! They are the common entities between the gut-brain connection that preserves memory. It is now believed that eating a healthy dose of dietary fiber regularly through wholesome meals provides enough dietary fiber that works with gut bacteria to modulate inflammation in the brain to avoid inflammatory injury to memory cells.

Japanese researchers studied[484] over three thousand seven hundred individuals for over thirty years. They found that, compared with those who eat the least amount of dietary fiber, those who eat the most dietary fiber have a twenty-five percent reduced risk of developing dementia. It is important to note that even in the 'highest' fiber intake group, many ate under twenty-five grams of fiber per day. In other words, in the research, the bar was kept low in what was considered high fiber intake, and nevertheless, there was still a twenty-five percent drop in dementia risk. It is possible that the observed difference would have been bigger than twenty-five percent if/when compared with a group eating north of thirty grams of dietary fiber per day. It is important to know that the researchers noted this twenty-five percent drop in risk even after further adjustment for potential mediators such as body mass index, systolic blood pressure, blood pressure medication use, serum total cholesterol, cholesterol-lowering medication, and diabetes.

P: Okay, we talked about fruit, vegetables, and fiber. Can you tell me if there is one food item I need to focus more on to prevent me from getting dementia like my dad did? What would that food be?

B: I am glad you asked me this. I have to say that that is the wrong place to start when we focus on one 'super-food' to fix one disease risk.

P: There goes all the money I spent on buying the superfoods I used to see in the news headlines!

B: Researchers in France conducted what is known as the "Three-city cohort study" [485] in the cities of Bordeaux, Dijon, and Montpellier in France. Over eight thousand people aged sixty-five and above were studied for four years. The primary intent of the study was to look at what they ate and how that impacted their risk of developing dementia. The researchers also verified this correlation to whether the individuals had a genetic tendency for Alzheimer's dementia or not. Among the diet variables the researchers were interested in was the connection between dementia risk, various dietary sources of fats, and fruit and vegetables.

Regardless of genetic tendencies to develop Alzheimer's dementia, there was a protective effect for eating fruit and vegetables that was statistically significant (twenty-eight percent drop in risk of dementia). Another group that showed a protective effect was eating omega-3-rich sources such as soy, walnut, and rapeseed oil (a whopping fifty-four percent drop in dementia risk). They also noted that eating omega-6 oils without eating enough fruit, vegetables, or omega-3 sources led to doubling the risk of developing dementia.

The researchers did an interesting analysis of whether there was any benefit if people did everything wrong except one good thing. In other words, these people ate more of one good thing (the "superfoods") to prevent dementia and ate unhealthy in all other aspects of their daily meals. This analysis showed that these people did not get any benefit from eating more of only one good food and letting other areas of their diet slide. This study confirmed and validated what other studies have shown for different aspects of our health. Eating more than one "superfood" and doing everything else unhealthy will not buy us good health. The research confirmed that combining dietary sources of omega-3 PUFA and antioxidants seems necessary for a protective effect against dementia.

P: Are you saying that the combination of ingredients in the meal matters more than one ingredient or portion size?

B: Correct! The meal pattern and mix of healthy ingredients for the day and the week is what has been shown to improve long-term health. There is no single super-food to improve our long-term health. Variety is key, the spice of life! By the way, your diet changes are helping me regulate your mood better[486, 487, 488, 489, 490] by releasing more of the 'lift me up' serotonin hormone[491] as they work with gut bacteria.[492, 493]

P: Yes, I could feel like the depression is leaving gradually[494, 495].

B: Correct. The diet changes that reduce sugars, fats and excess protein and increased dietary fiber and plant nutrients also help with anxiety[496, 497].

P: I remember the early days when Dad's decline began with his bone marrow not working well to produce blood cells.

B: Yes, the myelodysplasia was such a challenge.

P: Thank goodness we had a network of compassionate blood donors who donated blood for Dad yearly to keep him going. I love that the donor network was made of total strangers to Dad. The group members didn't know each other that well before connecting over Dad's need for regular blood transfusions. Now, they are family!

Alejandro - the first one to jump in for the blood donation, is a building contractor. I met him in a community fundraiser soccer match to benefit the local school that took a bad hit in a winter storm and needed repairs.

I was the goalie, and Alejandro was the defense. It was the day after Dad met with his hematologist to discuss his low blood counts. Alejandro signed up for a blood donation the day after the soccer game.

After interviewing at least four builders, Grace hired Alejandro for the extension in her house. He pulled in Grace to become a donor. He was inspired by the healthy state of Grace, reinforcing his conviction to follow his doctor's diet advice. The blood donor site team was more impressed with Grace and her hemoglobin levels.

Grace rents the house extension for River.

Jason told me how he does the annual tax return filling for River and in one of their conversations, she mentioned to him about looking for more blood donors for Dad.

Sarah is Jason's former colleague in the accounting world and they remained as good friends since her retirement.

Jen is Jason's niece.

Lauren is Jen's favorite staff at her regular coffee shop that she can't stop talking about.

Lauren and Iris are neighbors.

"Family tree"

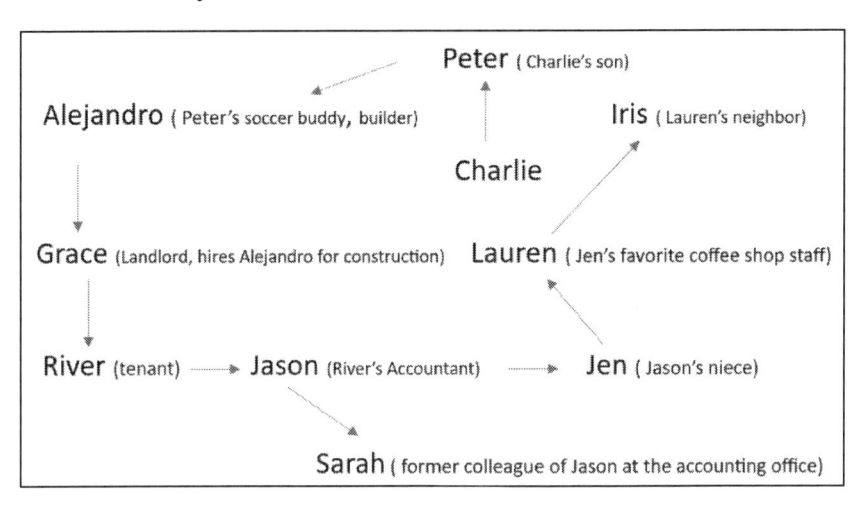

```
        Peter (Charlie's son)
              ↑
Alejandro (Peter's soccer buddy, builder)    Iris (Lauren's neighbor)
                        Charlie
   ↓
Grace (Landlord, hires Alejandro for construction)   Lauren (Jen's favorite coffee shop staff)
   ↓
River (tenant) → Jason (River's Accountant) → Jen (Jason's niece)
                    ↓
              Sarah (former colleague of Jason at the accounting office)
```

B: Family - not of blood-relation but connected by blood-donation.

Peter: It is still unbelievable! The support for the low blood cell count also served as the support I got for his decline due to dementia.

Miracles do happen! And to have the entire 'family' here during this day to visit Dad to bid farewell to him is so meaningful to Dad and me. The least I could do to show my gratitude is arrange for the meditation sessions for those visiting Dad during this weekend.

Talking about miracles reminds me of Iris, who is pregnant yet took the time and effort to travel to see Dad. I think she is next up on the schedule for the meditation session. Let me make sure she knows how to get to the meditation room in the herb garden.

I am definitely looking forward to our next conversation when I sit for meditation again. In the meantime, let's summarize what we talked about in this session:

> 1. Wholefood, plant-based diet combined with other lifestyle changes improves mild dementia from Alzheimer's disease.
> 2. Meditation improves memory and attention.
> 3. Avoiding sugary food and eating vegetables, whole grains, nuts, and seeds is the 401(K) future savings for memory cells.
> 4. Insulin resistance is bad for diabetes and dementia.
> 5. Long-term inflammation impacts memory. Inflammation is increased by excess calories that build visceral fat and injury to gut lining from high fats and sugars in food.
> 6. Eating healthy carbohydrates will not only help prevent diabetes but also reduce the risk of dementia.
> 7. Brain food is unprocessed carbohydrates. Dietary protein and fats can't get into the brain cells easily.
> 8. Genetic risk for dementia is overcome by eating more vegetables and fruit.
> 9. Memory protection from omega-3-rich sources such as soy, walnut, flax meal.

CHAPTER TEN
PRECIOUS MIRACLE: PREGNANCY

> Seven-word synopsis
> ***Wholefood plant meals amplify healthy pregnancy***

It is Iris's turn for the meditation session. She gives herself a few additional minutes in planning to get ready for this session. She knows that even simple activities and movements take extra effort and more time when you are carrying extra pounds for a good reason. That means even getting up from a reclined position can be awkward when your abdomen is in the way. Over the course of almost forty weeks of pregnancy, Iris has learned to always turn to her side from a reclined position before getting up in order to work around her full, curvy abdomen. Iris is at full-term in her first pregnancy. It is also her first successful pregnancy through in-vitro fertilization. Iris and her partner had been planning this pregnancy for nearly four years, and things have not always been smooth sailing along the way. They did agree on one thing: to move forward with the idea of having a family through pregnancy. Every decision after that has had its differences between the two of them requiring negotiation, some give and some take, and not always meeting half-way, but they made it work. The most difficult and challenging moments brought them closer in their relationship, especially after the first attempt with in-vitro fertilization didn't succeed. Naturally, the failed attempt also just added to the stress for the couple. And the stress factor didn't help the outcome of the second attempt at pregnancy[498].

Iris shifted to mindfulness meditation as one of her coping skills for managing stress[499, 500, 501] and worry about another failed attempt at pregnancy[502]. The mindfulness tools also help with getting centered during the process of working through their differences. Along with her learning of mindfulness meditation came additional awareness of paying attention to what she was consuming in terms of food and beverages. Mindful eating became part of the process of preparing for mindful conception. Her third attempt to get pregnant worked.

The timing of this visit to Peter's dad, Charlie, wasn't perfect, given that Iris is due to deliver the baby any day now. However, the bond she and other blood donors of Charlie have developed within the blood donation network group is strong. And it appeared that Charlie's mind-body-spirit was getting ready for transitioning from this physical world after two years of struggles with not being able to make blood cells in addition to the dementia that got progressively worse over the past eight years. The blood transfusions from the donor network that Peter built and nurtured kept the myelodysplasia disorder of not making enough blood cells manageable with multiple blood transfusions. However, dementia could not be kept in check. Iris didn't want to miss out on this opportunity to say goodbye to Charlie, so she made the effort to make it here for this gathering. Peter wanted to show his gratitude to all the blood donors who showed up to say goodbye to Charlie. Hence, the spa and meditation services that he made available to the visitors.

It didn't take long for Iris to get into meditation mode. It is a familiar mind-body space for her due to the recent years of mindfulness practice.

Body: What did you learn during your pregnancy?

Iris: In the beginning, my partner and I were anxious about the pregnancy process.

B: Do you want to talk more about what you learned about the anxiety you were feeling then and what you learned from it as you overcame it?

I: At a very fundamental level, being afraid or worried and, at the same time, trying to conceive a healthy offspring does not usually align well[503] - regardless of what form the living organism is in - whether it is a human or deer or ants or a bacterium. Response to fear diverts energy from the drive for procreating new life.

B: You are correct about the changes I feel now and then based on what the mind can incite. In the past, your fear and anxiety will set off what is called the fright/fight/flight response in the body, with our automatic nervous system instantly readying the body to deal with that situation that prompted the response: racing/pounding of the heart, eyes becoming alert and wide open, skin getting colder, blood pumping into the muscles of the legs which just picked up the pace of walking very quickly.

Every change I bring in instantaneously is geared toward readying the person for flight or fight. Wider eyes to take in as much visual information as possible, more quick-burning fuel in the form of glucose poured into the blood circulation, and more powerful and frequent impetus from the pump (fast, pounding heart beat) to push that fuel and oxygen toward the muscles that are going to require the fuel, wide opening of gates of blood vessels in the muscles to receive the fuel and oxygen, and diverting more fluids from other areas such as mouth and skin to give to the circulation feeding the muscles. The feeling of a dry mouth and cold skin due to the diversion of fluids to the muscles is not fun.

I: I know, we know. I have been there more than a few times!

B: When fear, worry, and concern are the dominant themes, I, the body, am too busy spending all my energy building up for the fright/flight/fight. This sets me up to divert energy from my focus and resource allocation for creating the environment for healthy conception. I am excited that you are ensuring that all your daily plant-based meal plans are well-balanced[504, 505, 506]. A "well-balanced vegetarian and vegan diets should be considered safe for the mother's health and for offspring during pregnancy and lactation."[507]

I: Let's hear what is behind the excitement.

B: Where do we start? A big one we dodged is the risk of a complication in pregnancy called 'pre-eclampsia', high blood pressure during pregnancy. Eating more plant-based meals, which are good sources of dietary fiber, magnesium, and potassium[508, 509], has been shown to protect against this complication that can be fatal for the mother and the baby. More than one in three strokes among pregnant mothers occur due to pre-eclampsia. Rarely, pre-eclampsia can lead to the placenta separating from the womb, basically closing all nutrition and oxygen to the fetus, threatening the life of the fetus as well as risking life-threatening (mother's life) bleeding from the uterus. Another way your plant-based eating style helped was to keep your pre-pregnancy weight within a normal range of body weight for your age and height[510] so that the risk of pre-eclampsia and high blood pressure was low[511, 512, 513, 514, 515] even before you conceived the baby.

I: I am happy that I also didn't gain excess weight during pregnancy.

B: Correct. That's another benefit of eating more plant-based meals that has been studied. Mothers who ate 'vegetarian' diets and were physically active were shown to avoid excess weight gain during pregnancy[516, 517]. Additionally, this, in turn, reduces their risk for pre-eclampsia.

Something else connected with excess weight gain during pregnancy is 'gestational diabetes,' an abnormal blood glucose problem that happens during pregnancy. Again, the way you were eating more plant-based meals[518, 519] with high dietary fiber reduced your risk of developing diabetes during pregnancy[520]. [521]Every 10-gram increment in daily intake of dietary fiber intake cuts the risk of gestational diabetes by 26%. When the part of me that receives your meal, i.e., your stomach, can only accommodate a finite amount of food for each meal, the proportion of the meal having dietary fiber makes a huge difference, especially because many foods commonly consumed such as all animal-derived food, processed grains and carbohydrates, and sugar have zero fiber. The meal becomes 'value-added' when most or all of the ingredients have dietary fiber[522, 523].

I: It is nice to hear your validation that I was on the right track, switching my diet three years ago when I was beginning to contemplate having a family.

I ensured I spoke with a registered dietitian to understand how to hit all the essential nutrient areas during my plant-based pregnancy. I tried my best to learn about nutrition and applied it to my daily menu. I just needed to get the best outcome possible for me and the baby.

B: You certainly did the right thing for the baby in your womb. You increased the chances of having the delivery closer to the due date instead of a premature birth, which can be risky for the baby. Your kind of diet, high in vegetables and fruits has been associated with reducing the risk of pre-term delivery[524]. This keeps the baby for the ideal duration inside the protected womb and a steady flow of food and oxygen through the umbilical cord.

Another way your diet is shown to protect the unborn baby is to limit any exposure to cancer-inducing chemicals[525]. A diet high in colorful fruits and vegetables and low in animal foods limits the amount of circulating cancer-inducing chemicals/toxins. Named 'genotoxins,' these chemicals bind to the DNA in the cell's genes and circulate in the blood that passes through the placenta to the unborn child. Scientists measure this by looking at the level of 'DNA adducts,' basically DNA bound to the cancer-inducing chemical. High vegetable and fruit intake has shown to have less of these 'DNA adducts' in umbilical blood[526]. It is important to note that the presence of these DNA adducts doesn't mean that the unborn baby *will* get cancer, but it does increase the chances of such an unfortunate outcome. Fetal cells are especially vulnerable because of the speed at which the cells multiply during the formation of different body systems within the embryo. A faster rate of cell multiplication inherently carries the risk of DNA breaks. DNA bound to cancer-inducing chemicals arriving through the placenta further increases the chance of DNA breaks. On the other hand, the colors in the colorful fruits and vegetables have what are called antioxidants protect against this.

I: I say, go vegetables!

B: Among the systems and organs that grow out of the embryo, one particular organ growing in the womb that is especially vulnerable to such DNA-adducts is the developing brain of the unborn child.

I: Brain tumors?

B: Correct. The cured meats[527] and smoked fish that were absent in your meals and the way you cut way back on pickled vegetables in your weekly meals - both these actions ensured that your exposure to *artificially added* nitrates/nitrites, and N-nitroso compounds (NOCs), shortly called 'nasty Ns' were minimal (note that the *naturally present* nitrates in leafy greens are not on this 'nasty Ns' list but is rather in the good list that helps our arteries stay open and healthy). Also, since you were eating at the lower end of the food chain for virtually all your meals except for New Year's dinner, the nitrites from ground water were not reaching your system through food at a high concentration and gets converted to carcinogenic nitrosamines as they would have for someone eating food from the higher end of the food chain (e.g., eating sausage, salami, bacon or cheese)[528]. These 'nasty Ns' are toxic to the growing fetal cells, especially the brain cells, since fetal brain cells lack the defense system to deal with nitrite exposure (alkyltransferase that repairs DNA adducts)[529].

B: The key to the way you are eating, which is virtually all plant-based meals, is that you are making sure you cover all your nutritional needs by focusing on the variety of the plant-foods that you are eating. The Vitamin B12 and folic acid supplement was a nice back-up insurance in the event that you didn't plan your meals well for a week.

I: The little extra effort I had to put in for the weekly meal planning is nothing compared with the benefits to me and the baby from eating this way. I only really had to make an effort for the first trimester. By the end of the fourth month, I had developed an eating routine that covered all my nutritional needs, and it had become second nature.

B: I remember you attending that session with the registered dietitian during the first month of the pregnancy. You had sections for calories, protein, calcium, iron, folic acid, Vitamin D, Vitamin B12, Choline, Iodine, and omega-3 fats.

I: I know. I had the key numbers stuck on the kitchen cabinet door. I know it so well that I can teach other women who are preparing for pregnancy.

B: Let's practice it now, can we?

I: Why not? Let's start with calories. According to the Dietary Reference Intakes (DRIs) and the Institute of Medicine (IOM), caloric necessities are no higher than the estimated energy requirement for non-pregnant women until the second trimester[530]. The extra energy requirement per day is 340 kcal in the second trimester and 452 kcal in the third trimester (IOM). You could meet that target of additional calories by adding two snacks throughout the course of the day.

B: Yes, I am so happy you have been adding those snacks between meals since the beginning of your second trimester. I love the taste of the Lemon Meringue Chia Pudding and how it helped our different parts and supplied nutrients to the baby. And I cannot forget the Peach Baked Oatmeal. And the delicious Garlicky Edamame Dip, which also added protein with the calcium from the tahini.

I: Correct. That's a good segue to practice sharing what I learned about additional protein requirements for months four to nine in pregnancy, regardless of what type of plant-based diet you are on, or not. Those who don't have a balanced meal are at higher risk of protein deficiency, especially during the second and third trimesters when additional dietary protein requirements exist. This is true for those who eat 100% plant-based, like me, or for someone who eats another way.

B: You did pay attention to adding more calories and ensuring that those additional calories were balanced with enough protein, healthy carbohydrates, and healthy omega-3 fats. That took care of the additional protein need, from my point of view, at the receiving end.

I: Yes, I made sure I increased the protein intake by 25 grams daily. I was told that would be an adequate increase to my baseline intake of 45 grams. Now, I am hitting 70 grams daily. This covers what the nutrition professionals recommend - that the mother needs to aim for a total protein intake that equals 1.1 g/kg of body weight daily.

B: The 'everything bagel crispy chickpeas' you were snacking on and the 'garlicky edamame dip' you chose for snacks made it easy to make up the additional need for protein. And, beyond these beans and legumes[531], how you had a balanced meal with vegetables, whole-grains, nuts, and seeds made sure you were hitting the target protein number for your pregnancy with all the essential amino-acid building-blocks without much sweat. It made me wonder what the fuss is about when people talk about protein when folks eat plant-based meals and are not even pregnant or have other such situations with a higher need for protein.

I: The balancing act has become easy with practice and repetition.

B: The other nutrient I hear a lot about when talking about plant-based meals and pregnancy is calcium. The experts recommend that vegetarians and vegans should consume 1200 to 1500 mg/day of calcium. Generally, plant protein does not create a loss of calcium in the urine like animal protein does, so, in that sense, this 1200 mg/ day of calcium allows for an extra buffer built into it since the calcium that comes into the body stays in without being lost in the urine.

I: I remember how the dietitians emphasized four things to reach my daily calcium goals.

1. Leafy greens with a little lemon squeezed onto them so that the Vitamin C in the lemon juice can pull enough calcium from the greens when they are being digested in my stomach.

2. Beans - different types, and this was also meeting my protein needs, so that was an efficient way of getting more than one nutrient need achieved through these choices – bringing down two apples from the tree with one stone!

3. Cup of fortified non-dairy milk

4. Sesame seeds, which is why I love the Lemon-Tahini Sauce for dressing my salads daily.

I: Reaching the calcium goal through my weekly meal plan became easier than I originally thought. What I found easy was that if I used the basic approach of eating a variety of foods from the various categories such as vegetables, whole-grains, beans/legumes, fruit nuts, and seeds - it appeared to cover the nutrient needs of my pregnancy. So far, my pre-natal visits have been positive, with a good report of health for me and the baby.

B: As you mentioned the seeds, it is hard for me to ignore mentioning the ground flax seeds that you add to your breakfast or salads daily. Just those two tablespoons cover your need for omega-3 healthy fats for you and the growing baby.

I: Flax has become a routine part of breaking-my-fast in the morning. Additionally, for omega-3 fats, I sometimes add Mungo beans[532], also known as Black gram (not to be confused with mung beans) to my soups and skip the flax on the days I am having the chia seed pudding since the chia seeds bring in the omega-3 fats. The omega-3 fats from leafy greens and walnuts that I eat are an extra bonus!

Also, with the amount of foliage, that is, leafy greens I eat daily, as well as the beans, fruits, nuts, seeds, and whole grains that are part of my diet, I cover the 600 micrograms of dietary folic acid equivalents I need daily during my pregnancy. Still, daily, I take the pre-natal vitamin with folic acid in it to cover for days I may not have planned the meals well, which can potentially happen when traveling. In those instances, I don't want to take a chance and miss out on meeting the daily requirement of folic acid because I know how much impact it can have on the baby. The neural-tube-defect in the baby's spinal cord from inadequate folic acid intake is totally preventable[533].

B: Correct, unnecessary trouble, really. I also appreciate the new flavoring made out of kelp that you are adding to your soups and salads. That is guaranteeing the 220 micrograms of iodine that I am looking for daily for you and your baby, given that you use very minimal iodized salt for your meals.

I: Over the years, I have realized that flavoring my meals with herbs and spices is more than enough to flavor them without relying on salt.

B: I am also very happy you alternate between lima beans and edamame beans in your weekly routine. Those beans, along with your intake of shiitake mushrooms, a variety of vegetables and fruit, and the routine sprinkling of wheat germ in your breakfast - all this is making sure I am getting the 450 micrograms of Choline daily for the baby and us.

I: Luckily, the fundamental formula for covering many nutrient needs in pregnancy is that I have variety in the sources of my food ingredients.

With a gentle transition, Iris ended her meditation session. She was reminiscing about the fond conversation she had had earlier in the day with Charlie at his bedside when she saw the hospice nurse Kim coming out of Charlie's room. 'He is struggling to breathe from the aspiration. We are honoring Charlie's wishes to focus on keeping him comfortable", said Kim as she went to grab the next dose of comfort care medicine for Charlie.

Iris senses it could be a matter of just a few hours and is grateful she made the trip to see Charlie before he passes.

It was then she noticed that she had wet her dress, with the effect traveling all along down her legs to her heels. 'I have never had a urinary accident before' - her mind started to analyze and think back if she had overlooked any sign of urinary infection such as a burning in her urine. Her mind was pulled back to reality by the squeeze she started to feel in her pelvis. Then it dawned on her. She picked up the phone and called her partner. After the first ring, the call was answered.

"My water just broke. I think I am starting to have contractions", said Iris with a nervous excitement in her voice.

> **Summary of discussion in this session:**
>
> 1. Fear and worry divert energy from the drive for procreating new life and is associated with infertility.
> 2. Mindfulness meditation helps cope/manage stress.
> 3. Well-balanced wholefood, plant-based diet is safe during pregnancy and also protects against weight gain during pregnancy and pre-eclampsia.
> 3. Every 10-gram increment in daily intake of dietary fiber intake cuts the risk of gestational diabetes by 26%.
> 4. Diets high in colorful fruits and vegetables and low in animal foods limit the amount of circulating cancer-inducing 'genotoxins' in umbilical cord.
> 5. 'Nasty Ns' are toxic to growing fetal cells, especially brain cells. They are artificially added nitrates/nitrites and N-nitroso compounds (NOCs) from sausage, salami, bacon, some cheese types, smoked fish and pickled vegetables. Nutrition labels list the toxic *added* nitrites/nitrates as 'sodium nitrite' / 'potassium nitrate'.
> 6. Pregnant mothers need to aim for a total protein intake that equals 1.1 g/kg of body weight daily. This is easy to do with plant foods.
> 7. Healthy pregnancy using wholefood plant-based nutrition requires attention to meal planning that covers the daily requirements of calories, protein, calcium, iron, folic acid, Vitamin D, Vitamin B12, Choline, Iodine, and omega-3 fats.

RECIPES

BREAKFAST — 187

- Lemon Meringue Chia Pudding — 188
- Kale and Mushroom Omelet — 191
- Anti-inflammatory Mango Berry Smoothie — 194
- Southwestern Tofu Scramble and Oil-free Crispy Hash Browns — 196
- Peach Baked Oatmeal — 201
- Savory Grits with Oat-walnut Sausage Patties — 204

SAUCES + DRESSINGS — 208

- Herby Ranch Dressing — 209
- Lemon-Tahini Sauce — 211
- Go-To Vinaigrette — 213
- "Cheesy" Sauce — 214
- Zesty Peanut Sauce — 216
- Mango Citrus Dressing — 218

LUNCH + DINNER — 219

- Smoky BBQ Tempeh Sheet Pan Dinner with Roasted Vegetables — 220
- Sweet Potato Quesadillas with Purple Cabbage Slaw — 223
- Creamy Cauliflower Alfredo Pasta — 227
- Quick Thai Salad with Zesty Peanut Dressing — 230
- Simple Bean Burgers — 232
- Chickpea of the Sea Salad — 235
- Root Vegetable Soup with Citrusy Arugula Salad — 237
- Red Lentil Curry — 240
- Sesame Noodle Bowl — 242

Slow Cooker Tuscan White Bean Stew	244
Ultimate Chopped Salad	246
Tofu Poke Bowl	248

SNACKS + DESSERTS — 250

One Bowl Oatmeal Cookies	251
Stuffed Dates	253
Garlicky Edamame Dip	255
Cacao Mousse with Fresh Berries	257
Everything Bagel Crispy Chickpeas	259
Cheesy Kale Chips	261
Seasonal Fruit Crumble	263

BREAKFAST

Lemon Meringue Chia Pudding

Serves 4

Nutrition Info Per Serving

- ❖ Calories: 346
- ❖ Carbohydrates: 31g
- ❖ Fiber: 11g
- ❖ Total Fat: 21g
- ❖ Sat Fat: 5g
- ❖ Protein: 13g
- ❖ Sodium: 75mg

Description Notes:

- Chia seeds have multiple health benefits because they are high in Omega-3 fats (healthy, anti-inflammatory fat), dietary fiber, and minerals.
- A great make-ahead recipe for grab-and-go breakfast, snack, or even dessert
- Can make up to 5 days ahead (may need to stir and add more plant-based milk because it will thicken over time)

Ingredients:

- 3 cups unsweetened plant-based milk
- ½ cup chia seeds
- 1 tablespoon maple syrup or date syrup
- 2 tablespoons lemon juice
- ¼ teaspoon vanilla extract

- ¼ cup sliced almonds
- 2 tablespoons unsweetened, flaked, toasted coconut
- 2 cups strawberries, sliced

Instructions:

1. In a medium bowl, whisk together the plant-based milk, chia seeds, maple syrup or date syrup, lemon juice, and vanilla extract.
2. Let the mixture sit for about 15 minutes, and then whisk again. Cover and refrigerate overnight or for at least 8 hours.
3. In the morning, stir the mixture and add plant-based milk to adjust to the desired consistency. Divide into four bowls, and top with almonds, coconut, and strawberries.

Notes:

- Any unsweetened plant-based milk will work. Try soy, almond, or oat milk.
- Substitute any nuts or seeds in place of the sliced almonds. Try walnuts or pecans. For a nut-free version, try pumpkin seeds.
- If you aim to reduce calories and saturated fat, reduce the amount of coconut flakes you use or replace them with extra fruit.
- Substitute any fruit for the strawberries. Try blueberries, chopped apples, or figs.

- Make up to 5 days in advance. The mixture will thicken as time passes, so you may need to stir in additional plant-based milk.

Kale and Mushroom Omelet

Serves 2

Nutrition Info Per Serving

- ❖ Calories: 305
- ❖ Carbohydrates: 44g
- ❖ Fiber: 11g
- ❖ Total Fat: 6g
- ❖ Sat Fat: 1g
- ❖ Protein: 19g
- ❖ Sodium: 485mg

Description Notes:

- Chickpea flour is a protein-rich ingredient for breakfast with dietary fiber and zero cholesterol.
- Kale and mushrooms are both good sources of iron, with kale adding antioxidants and phytonutrients.
- Nutritional yeast adds an "umami" flavor.

Ingredients:

- 2 teaspoons walnut oil (optional, see instructions)
- 1 cup chickpea flour
- 1 tablespoon ground flaxseed
- ¼ teaspoon salt
- ½ teaspoon garlic powder
- ½ teaspoon onion powder
- ¼ teaspoon turmeric

- 2 tablespoons nutritional yeast
- ¼ teaspoon baking soda
- 1 cup water
- ½ cup kale, chopped
- ½ red onion, chopped
- ½ cup mushrooms (cremini, button, or any other variety you like), sliced
- Salsa (optional)
- Avocado slices (optional)

Instructions:

1. Preheat a skillet over medium heat.
2. In a bowl, combine the chickpea flour, ground flaxseed, salt, garlic powder, onion powder, turmeric, nutritional yeast, and baking soda.
3. Make a well in the center of the dry ingredients, and slowly add water while stirring. Stir until no dry spots remain in the batter.
4. Add a drizzle of oil to the skillet (or even better, skip the oil and use a non-toxic, non-stick skillet), and pour half of the batter into the skillet. Sprinkle with half of the chopped kale, onion, and mushrooms. Let cook for 4-5 minutes or until the omelet begins to cook through.
5. Carefully flip the omelet and cook for a few more minutes until it easily releases from the pan. Remove the cooked

omelet from the skillet, and repeat with the remaining batter.

6. Serve topped with salsa and avocado slices.

Notes:

- To prevent sticking, use a good non-stick skillet or oil to coat the skillet.

- Replace the salt with black salt to create an egg-like smell and taste. Black salt has a sulfurous smell and taste that lends the perfect eggy qualities to this dish.

- Season this omelet with any of your favorite spices. Add chili powder and cumin for a Southwestern flavor, or try parsley, chives, and tarragon for a French flavor.

- Any vegetables are fair game for this recipe! Swap the kale, onion, and mushrooms for sliced peppers, shaved Brussels sprouts, arugula, or whatever you have. Leftover roasted vegetables also work wonderfully.

Anti-inflammatory Mango Berry Smoothie

Serves 1

Nutrition Info Per Serving

- ❖ Calories: 450
- ❖ Carbohydrates: 53g
- ❖ Fiber: 13g
- ❖ Total Fat: 19g
- ❖ Sat Fat: 2g
- ❖ Protein: 20g
- ❖ Sodium: 271mg

Description Notes:

- This recipe has a mix of anti-inflammatory ingredients like berries, greens, flax, and turmeric.
- Cruciferous vegetables such as cauliflower are a vital addition to prevent cancer.
- Frozen cauliflower makes this smoothie decadently creamy - you won't even taste it!
- A pinch of black pepper greatly enhances turmeric's absorption into the cells.

Ingredients:

- ½ cup frozen cauliflower florets
- ½ cup frozen mixed berries
- ¾ cup frozen mango
- ½ cup baby spinach

- 1 banana
- 2 tablespoons ground flaxseed
- ¼ teaspoon turmeric powder
- Pinch of black pepper
- 2 cups plant-based milk

Instructions:

1. Combine all ingredients in a blender. Blend until smooth, stopping to stir as needed.

Notes:

- The spinach can be swapped for any leafy green you have. Try kale or romaine.
- Instead of flaxseeds, try chia seeds or hemp seeds. All of these nutritious seeds give this smoothie an omega-3 boost.
- To adjust the smoothie's consistency, add more or less plant-based milk during blending.
- Meal prep tip: Pre-portion smoothie ingredients into individual bags or containers. Make enough grab-and-go bags for the week and store them in the freezer. When you're ready to make the smoothie, simply pull out a pre-portioned bag, dump it into the blender, blend, and go!

Southwestern Tofu Scramble and Oil-free Crispy Hash Browns

Serves 4

Tofu Scramble Nutrition Info Per Serving

- ❖ Calories: 112
- ❖ Carbohydrates: 7g
- ❖ Fiber: 3g
- ❖ Total Fat: 5g
- ❖ Sat Fat: 1g
- ❖ Protein: 12g
- ❖ Sodium: 200mg

Hash Brown Nutrition Info Per Serving

- ❖ Calories: 167
- ❖ Carbohydrates: 38g
- ❖ Fiber: 5g
- ❖ Total Fat: 0g
- ❖ Sat Fat: 0g
- ❖ Protein: 4g
- ❖ Sodium: 159mg

Description Notes:

- A hearty, savory breakfast that could be eaten as is or wrapped up in tortillas for breakfast tacos or burritos.

- Tofu is made of soybeans (also called edamame beans) through coagulation using natural calcium in the form of gypsum. It is a high-value food for nutrients such as phytoestrogens that protect against cancers, especially breast cancer - both the hormone-receptor positive and negative types. It is also a rich source of protein that packs all essential amino acids in one food and is a high course of dietary fiber and calcium.

INGREDIENTS

- 4 potatoes (or 4 cups of frozen shredded hash browns)
- ½ teaspoon black pepper
- ½ teaspoon salt
- ½ teaspoon of onion powder
- ½ teaspoon of garlic powder
- 1 (14-ounce) block of firm tofu
- 1 tablespoon tamari/low-sodium soy sauce
- 1 tablespoon nutritional yeast
- 1 teaspoon turmeric powder
- ½ teaspoon chili powder
- ½ teaspoon cumin powder
- 4 cups baby spinach
- ½ cup low-sodium salsa
- Hot sauce (optional)

INSTRUCTIONS

For the Hash Browns:

1. Prepare the potatoes. Shred potatoes using a food processor with a grater attachment or a handheld grater.
2. Preheat oven to 400 degrees F and line a baking sheet with parchment paper. Spread the potato shreds onto the prepared baking sheet in an even layer. Sprinkle with onion

powder, garlic powder, pepper, and salt, and toss to coat. Bake for 10-15 minutes until the underside of the hash browns gets brown and crispy. Flip the hash browns and bake for another 5 minutes on the second side until crispy.

For the Tofu Scramble:

1. Drain and press tofu between two layers of paper towels or dish towels to remove as much water as possible.

2. Crumble the tofu with your hands into a small bowl. Add tamari/soy sauce, nutritional yeast, turmeric, chili powder, and cumin, and lightly stir until the tofu is evenly covered.

3. Heat a skillet over medium heat and add the tofu mixture. Cook, stirring frequently, until the tofu is heated through and enough water has evaporated to give it the consistency of scrambled eggs. Just before the tofu is done, add the spinach. When spinach is wilted, remove from heat.

4. Serve tofu scramble with hash browns. Top with salsa and hot sauce.

Notes:

- Replace the salt with black salt ("Kala namak") to create an egg-like smell and taste. Black salt has a sulfurous smell and taste that lends the perfect eggy qualities to this scramble.

- If you don't have spinach, any leafy green will work. Try kale, swiss chard, or arugula.

- Add sauteed vegetables or leftover roasted vegetables to the scramble for an extra veggie boost.

- Transform this recipe into breakfast tacos or burritos by wrapping it in a whole-grain tortilla.

Peach Baked Oatmeal

Serves 5

Nutrition Info Per Serving

- Calories: 404
- Carbohydrates: 59g
- Fiber: 7g
- Total Fat: 14g
- Sat Fat: 3g
- Protein: 12g
- Sodium: 149mg

Description Notes:

- This a wonderful oat recipe for anyone who doesn't like the texture of traditional cooked oatmeal
- It can easily be made ahead and reheated in the oven or microwave
- Oats are high in a dietary fiber called beta-glucan fiber, which works with gut bacteria to create short-chain fatty acids that stimulate the secretion of appetite-regulating hormones.
- Oats are also good protein, magnesium, thiamine, and zinc sources.

INGREDIENTS

- 2½ cups old-fashioned oats
- 1 teaspoon baking powder
- ½ cup walnuts

- 2½ cups plant-based milk
- 1 teaspoon vanilla extract
- ½ cup unsweetened applesauce
- ¼ cup maple syrup or date syrup
- 3-4 peaches, pitted and sliced

INSTRUCTIONS

1. Preheat oven to 450 degrees F and lightly oil a 2-quart casserole dish (or skip the oil and line the dish with parchment paper).
2. In a large bowl, combine oats, baking powder, and walnuts.
3. Add milk, applesauce, maple or date syrup, vanilla extract, and sliced peaches. Stir until evenly combined.
4. Pour the mixture into the prepared casserole dish and gently smooth the surface. Bake for 45 minutes or until browned and bubbly around the edges.
5. Cool at least 5 minutes before slicing.
6. Serve topped with a plant-based milk splash, a nut butter dollop, and extra fruit.

Notes

- Substitute any nuts or seeds in place of the walnuts. Try pecans, almonds, or macadamia nuts. For a nut-free version, try pumpkin seeds.
- Any unsweetened plant-based milk will work. Try soy, almond, or oat milk.

- Substitute any fruit for the peaches. Try mixed berries, chopped apples, pears, or bananas.
- Sprinkle hemp, flax, or chia seeds over the top before baking for an added nutrient boost.
- You can bake these in a cupcake pan to make individual oatmeal cups that are great for traveling.

Savory Grits with Oat-walnut Sausage Patties

Serves 4

Savory Grits Nutrition Info Per Serving

- ❖ Calories: 162
- ❖ Carbohydrates: 31g
- ❖ Fiber: 4g
- ❖ Total Fat: 2g
- ❖ Sat Fat: 0g
- ❖ Protein: 5g
- ❖ Sodium: 148mg

Sausage Patties Nutrition Info Per Serving

- ❖ Calories: 246
- ❖ Carbohydrates: 13g
- ❖ Fiber: 4g
- ❖ Total Fat: 21g
- ❖ Sat Fat: 2g
- ❖ Protein: 6g
- ❖ Sodium: 54mg

Description Notes:

- This recipe is perfect for those looking to change their routine from porridge with fruit/nuts to something savory for breakfast.

- The sausage patties in this recipe are a wholefood alternative to processed faux meats/sausages high in sodium and processed ingredients. Both walnuts and flax that make up the sausage patties are high in anti-inflammatory omega-3 fats.

- Walnut oil may not have the same negative effects on arterial lining as other vegetable oils.

Savory Grits Ingredients

- 2 cups low-sodium vegetable broth
- 1 cup stone-ground cornmeal grits or polenta
- ½ teaspoon salt
- ⅛ teaspoon smoked paprika
- ¼ cup chopped scallions

Oat-walnut Sausage Patties Ingredients

- 1 tablespoon ground flaxseed
- 3 tablespoons water
- 1 cup walnuts
- 1/2 cup rolled oats
- 3 teaspoons walnut oil, divided (skip if using air fyer)
- 1 teaspoon maple syrup or date syrup
- 4 drops liquid smoke
- 1 teaspoon fennel seeds
- ½ teaspoon dried sage
- ½ teaspoon dried thyme
- Salt and pepper to taste

Savory Grits Instructions

1. In a saucepan, bring the vegetable broth to a boil.
2. Add the salt and smoked paprika, then slowly whisk in the grits.
3. Lower heat to a gentle simmer and cook for 15 minutes, stirring grits every few minutes until they are thick and creamy.
4. Remove from heat and stir in scallions.

Oat-walnut Sausage Patties Instructions

1. Prepare "flax egg": Combine ground flaxseed and water in a small bowl. Let sit for 5 minutes to thicken.
2. In a food processor, add all ingredients and pulse until well combined.
3. Scooping 1 heaping tablespoon of the sausage mixture at a time, shape the mixture into patties. Wetting your fingers will help form patties and prevent the mixture from sticking to your hands.
4. Heat walnut oil (optional) on a non-toxic, non-stick skillet over medium heat. Add patties to the hot pan. Cook for 2-3 minutes on each side or until brown. Alternatively, skip oil if using air fryer)
5. Top bowls of warm Savory Grits with crisp sausage patties, and enjoy.

Notes:

- Get creative with your Savory Grits toppings. Chopped herbs like cilantro, rosemary, or thyme would all be delicious options.

- Make-ahead option: freeze the uncooked sausage patties on a sheet pan. Once frozen, store in an air-tight container. When you're ready to cook them, remove them from the freezer and cook in a hot skillet according to the instructions. The frozen patties will take a little longer to cook fully.

- Enjoy the Oat-walnut Sausage Patties paired with the Tofu Scramble for a fresh breakfast combination.

- If you can access an air-fryer, you can make the patties without oil.

SAUCES + DRESSINGS

Herby Ranch Dressing

4 servings

Nutrition Info Per Serving

- ❖ Calories: 145
- ❖ Carbohydrates: 6g
- ❖ Fiber: 4g
- ❖ Total Fat: 14g
- ❖ Sat Fat: 12g
- ❖ Protein: 2g
- ❖ Sodium: 154mg

Description Notes:

- A healthy take on a classic dressing.
- It can be used as a dressing, dip, or sauce.

Ingredients:

- 1 cup unsweetened plain non-dairy yogurt
- Juice from 1 lemon
- 1 teaspoon white wine vinegar
- 2 cloves garlic
- 2 teaspoons fresh dill
- 2 teaspoons fresh parsley
- 2 teaspoons fresh chives
- ¼ teaspoon salt
- ¼ teaspoon black pepper

Instructions:

1. Add all ingredients to a deep bowl or jar and whisk until well combined. Store in an air-tight container in the refrigerator for up to 5 days.

Notes:

- This dressing makes a delicious dip for raw veggies and whole grain crackers and a perfect sauce to drizzle on roasted vegetables, tofu, or grain bowls.

Lemon-Tahini Sauce

4 servings

Nutrition Info Per Serving

- ❖ Calories: 131
- ❖ Carbohydrates: 6g
- ❖ Fiber: 2g
- ❖ Total Fat: 11g
- ❖ Sat Fat: 1g
- ❖ Protein: 5g
- ❖ Sodium: 153mg

Description Notes:

- Tahini is a sesame seed paste and is a good source of calcium.

Ingredients:

- 1/3 cup tahini
- Juice of 1 lemon
- ¼ cup nutritional yeast
- 1 garlic clove, peeled
- ¼ teaspoon salt
- ¼ cup water
- Chili pepper flakes (optional)

Instructions:

1. Combine all ingredients in a food processor or blender and blend until smooth. Slowly add more water as needed to

reach the desired consistency (a light creamy dressing consistency for salads or a thicker consistency for a dip).

Notes:

- Try different spices or flavor combinations in this base recipe.
- For a different take, use lime juice instead of lemon juice.

Go-To Vinaigrette

2 servings

Nutrition Info Per Serving

- ❖ Calories: 42
- ❖ Carbohydrates: 8g
- ❖ Fiber: 1g
- ❖ Total Fat: 0g
- ❖ Sat Fat: 0g
- ❖ Protein: 1g
- ❖ Sodium: 189mg

Description Notes:

- A very simple oil-free dressing to whip up any time.

Ingredients:

- ¼ cup balsamic vinegar
- ¼ cup water
- 1 tablespoon Dijon mustard
- 1 tablespoon salt-free Italian seasoning blend
- ½ teaspoon garlic powder
- Salt and pepper to taste

Instructions:

1. Combine all ingredients in a jar and shake until combined.

"Cheesy" Sauce

4 servings

Nutrition Info Per Serving

- ❖ Calories: 56
- ❖ Carbohydrates: 11g
- ❖ Fiber: 2g
- ❖ Total Fat: 0g
- ❖ Sat Fat: 0g
- ❖ Protein: 3g
- ❖ Sodium: 205mg

Description Notes:

- This is a crowd-pleaser! It's like a queso dip or nacho cheese sauce.
- The potato and carrot give it a creamy texture without the added fat.

Ingredients:

- 1 Yukon gold potato, diced
- 1 carrot, diced
- ⅓ cup nutritional yeast
- ½ cup water
- ½ teaspoon cumin
- ¼ teaspoon salt
- 2 tablespoons low-sodium salsa
- ⅛ teaspoon garlic powder

Instructions:

1. Put the diced potatoes and carrots in a saucepan. Add enough water so that about one-third of the vegetables are submerged. Cover, heat over medium-high, and steam until the potatoes and carrots are tender. They should fall apart when pierced with a fork.

2. Combine all ingredients in a blender until completely smooth and creamy. Slowly add more water as needed to reach the desired consistency.

Notes:

- Enjoy this as a queso-like dip or sauce for pasta, bowls, or tacos.

Zesty Peanut Sauce

4 servings

Nutrition Info Per Serving

- ❖ Calories: 137
- ❖ Carbohydrates: 6g
- ❖ Fiber: 1g
- ❖ Total Fat: 11g
- ❖ Sat Fat: 2g
- ❖ Protein: 6g
- ❖ Sodium: 323mg

Description Notes:

- A go-to sauce for dipping, drizzling, and pouring.

Ingredients

- 1/3 cup peanut butter
- 2 tablespoons tamari/low-sodium soy sauce
- 2 teaspoons sesame oil (optional)
- 2 teaspoons rice vinegar
- Juice of ½ a lime
- 1/2 cup water
- 1/2 teaspoon maple syrup or date syrup
- 1 teaspoon grated ginger

Instructions

1. Combine all ingredients and whisk together until smooth. Alternatively, blend in a food processor or blender.

Notes:

- Allergic to peanuts? Use cashew butter or tahini paste instead of peanut butter.
- Mix this sauce with extra rice vinegar to transform it into a dressing.

Mango Citrus Dressing

4 servings

Nutrition Info Per Serving

- ❖ Calories: 95
- ❖ Carbohydrates: 8g
- ❖ Fiber: 4g
- ❖ Total Fat: 7g
- ❖ Sat Fat: 1g
- ❖ Protein: 1g
- ❖ Sodium: 55mg

Description Notes:

- A sweet addition to savory salads and bowls

Ingredients

- 1 avocado
- ½ cup chopped mango, fresh or frozen, thawed
- Juice of 1 lime
- ½ cup fresh basil leaves or fresh cilantro leaves
- ½ cup water
- Salt and pepper to taste

Instructions

1. Combine all ingredients in a food processor or blender and blend until smooth. Drizzle and enjoy!

LUNCH + DINNER

Smoky BBQ Tempeh Sheet Pan Dinner with Roasted Vegetables

Serves 4

Nutrition Info Per Serving

- ❖ Calories: 271
- ❖ Carbohydrates: 63g
- ❖ Fiber: 7g
- ❖ Total Fat: 1g
- ❖ Sat Fat: 0g
- ❖ Protein: 5g
- ❖ Sodium: 736mg

Description Notes:

- The simplicity of using one pan for protein and vegetables in this dish results in fewer dishes to wash.
- Tempeh is the same as tofu, except it is fermented, adding enhanced benefits to keep the friendly bacteria in our gut healthy and thriving.
- Tempeh has the same benefits of cancer protection offered by tofu described on page 196.
- This recipe is packed with fiber from sweet potatoes, corn, and Brussels sprouts.

Ingredients:

- 2 sweet potatoes, cut into ½ inch cubes
- 1 cup corn kernels, fresh or frozen
- 2 cups Brussels sprouts, trimmed and halved

- 1 tablespoon walnut oil (optional)
- 1 teaspoon smoked paprika
- ½ teaspoon cumin
- ½ teaspoon garlic powder
- ½ teaspoon salt
- 1 (8-ounce) block tempeh, cut into ½ inch cubes
- ¾ cup no added sugar barbecue sauce, plus an additional ½ cup for serving

Instructions:

1. Marinate the tempeh: toss cubed tempeh with barbecue sauce in a shallow dish. Cover and refrigerate for at least 30 minutes or overnight.
2. Preheat the oven to 425 degrees F. Whisk together oil (optional), paprika, cumin, garlic powder, and salt in a large bowl. Add cubed sweet potatoes, corn, and halved Brussels sprouts. Toss to coat.
3. Spread the vegetables in a single layer on a sheet pan, reserving ⅓ of the space on the pan for the tempeh. Spread the marinated tempeh onto the remaining ⅓ of the sheet pan. Bake for 30 minutes or until everything is golden brown.
4. Serve with additional barbecue sauce for dipping.

Notes:

- To make this a heartier meal, serve with a side of cooked grains like brown rice, quinoa, or farro.

- Want to switch up the plant-based protein? Try a can of chickpeas (drained and rinsed) in place of the tempeh.

- Experiment with different vegetables like new potatoes, broccoli florets, or parsnips.

- Get creative with different sauces. "Cheesy" Sauce (p. 214) and Zesty Peanut Sauce (p. 216) are both delicious ways to reinvent this sheet pan meal.

Sweet Potato Quesadillas with Purple Cabbage Slaw

Serves 8

Quesadilla Nutrition Info Per Serving

- ❖ Calories: 230
- ❖ Carbohydrates: 44g
- ❖ Fiber: 11g
- ❖ Total Fat: 2g
- ❖ Sat Fat: 0g
- ❖ Protein: 12g
- ❖ Sodium: 616mg

Cabbage Slaw Nutrition Info Per Serving

- ❖ Calories: 17
- ❖ Carbohydrates: 4g
- ❖ Fiber: 1g
- ❖ Total Fat: 0g
- ❖ Sat Fat: 0g
- ❖ Protein: 1g
- ❖ Sodium: 153

Description Notes:

- This recipe is loaded with flavor and antioxidants added by sweet potatoes, purple cabbage, black beans, and salsa.
- This dish is kid friendly.

Cabbage Slaw Ingredients

- 2 cups purple cabbage, shredded
- 1 red onion, thinly sliced

- ¼ cup fresh cilantro, minced
- Juice of 1 lime
- ¼ cup apple cider vinegar
- 1 teaspoon chili powder
- 1 teaspoon cumin
- ½ teaspoon salt
- ½ teaspoon black pepper

Quesadilla Ingredients

- 2 large sweet potatoes, cubed (no need to peel)
- ½ cup low-sodium salsa
- 1 tablespoon chili powder
- Juice of one lime
- ¼ cup nutritional yeast
- 1 (15-ounce) can low-sodium black beans, drained and rinsed
- ½ teaspoon salt
- ½ teaspoon black pepper
- 8 (10-inch) whole grain or sprouted grain tortillas

Instructions

For the Slaw:

1. In a large bowl, combine the cabbage, onion, and cilantro.

2. Whisk together the lime juice, vinegar, chili powder, cumin, salt, and pepper in a small bowl. Pour the dressing over the cabbage mixture. Stir until completely coated.

3. Refrigerate overnight or for at least 30 minutes to allow the slaw to marinate.

For the Quesadillas:

1. Put the cubed sweet potatoes in a saucepan with enough water to cover. Bring to a boil, reduce heat, cover, and simmer until fork-tender. Drain.

2. Transfer cooked and drained sweet potatoes to a mixing bowl. Add salsa, chili powder, lime juice, and nutritional yeast. With a fork, smash and mix until well combined. For a smoother filling, smash the sweet potatoes into a puree. For more texture, leave the sweet potatoes slightly chunky. Fold in the black beans. Add salt and pepper.

3. Heat a grill or grill pan over medium heat. Spread a heaping ½ cup of the sweet potato mixture onto one tortilla. Place a second tortilla on top and press it down gently to form one quesadilla. Repeat this with the remaining tortillas to create 4 quesadillas.

4. Place each quesadilla on the heated grill and cook for about 3 minutes on each side until golden brown and grill marks form.

To serve

1. Slice the quesadillas into triangles and serve with a heaping scoop of slaw.

Notes:

- Try different beans like pinto beans, kidney beans, or lentils.

- Serve with "Cheesy" Sauce (p. 214) to make these quesadillas extra special.

- This quesadilla filling also makes an excellent filling for enchiladas or tacos.

Creamy Cauliflower Alfredo Pasta

Serves 8

Nutrition Info Per Serving

- ❖ Calories: 411
- ❖ Carbohydrates: 58g
- ❖ Fiber: 3g
- ❖ Total Fat: 16g
- ❖ Sat Fat: 3g
- ❖ Protein: 17g
- ❖ Sodium: 211mg

Description Notes:

- The recipe trades dairy for a cauliflower-based, high-fiber, low-fat sauce to increase the abundance of anti-cancer compounds such as sulforaphanes and indole-3-carbinol.

Ingredients

- 1 head of cauliflower
- 4 cloves garlic, peeled
- Salt and pepper to taste
- Pinch of nutmeg
- 1 cup plain unsweetened soymilk
- 16 ounces bean pasta or whole wheat pasta
- Plant-based Parmesan:
    - 2 cups raw cashews
    - ¼ cup nutritional yeast

- ½ teaspoon salt

Instructions

Prepare the Plant-based Parmesan:

1. Combine all ingredients in a food processor or blender and pulse until a fine, parmesan-like texture forms. Set aside.

Prepare the pasta and sauce:

1. Prepare the pasta according to the package directions.
2. While the pasta is cooking, cut cauliflower into florets. Steam cauliflower in a saucepan until tender enough to easily pierce with a fork. Transfer steamed cauliflower to a blender or food processor and add garlic, salt, pepper, nutmeg, and soymilk. Blend until completely smooth, adding more milk to thin it out. Stir in the Plant-based Parmesan.
3. Drain the pasta and return it to the pot. Add the Alfredo Sauce and gently toss the pasta to coat.
4. Serve with a side salad or a side of steamed or roasted vegetables.

Notes:

- This pasta dish is even more delicious with steamed broccoli florets.
- Bump up the protein of this meal by folding in cooked chickpeas or white beans.

- Substitute the cashews for sunflower seeds in the Plant-based Parmesan for a cashew-free version.
- Substitute the cashews for sunflower seeds in the Plant-based Parmesan for a nut-free version.
- The Plant-based Parmesan also makes a delicious topping for other dishes, including soups, grain bowls, and salads. It can be stored in the refrigerator for up to two weeks.

Quick Thai Salad with Zesty Peanut Dressing

Serves 1

Nutrition Info Per Serving

- ❖ Calories: 246
- ❖ Carbohydrates: 22g
- ❖ Fiber: 7g
- ❖ Total Fat: 13g
- ❖ Sat Fat: 2g
- ❖ Protein: 14g
- ❖ Sodium: 375mg

Notes:

- This recipe packs a punch with loads of plant protein from snap peas, bean sprouts, and edamame.
- This meal is filled with raw veggies that supply dietary fiber to benefit us and the friendly bacteria in our gut.

Ingredients

- 1 cup romaine, shredded
- ½ cup snap peas, roughly chopped
- 1 carrot, sliced into matchsticks
- ¼ cup bean sprouts
- ½ cup edamame beans
- 1 serving Peanut Sauce (p. 216)
- 2 teaspoons rice vinegar

Instructions:

1. Thin Peanut Sauce with rice vinegar, whisking until it reaches a pourable consistency.
2. Combine all ingredients in a large bowl and toss with dressing. Enjoy immediately.

Notes:

- Toss in whatever veggies you have on hand! Anything goes with this salad.
- Sprinkle with chopped peanuts or cashews for extra crunch.
- To make this salad heartier, add cooked and cooled brown rice noodles.

Simple Bean Burgers

Makes 8 patties

Nutrition Info Per Serving

- ❖ Calories: 70
- ❖ Carbohydrates: 12g
- ❖ Fiber: 4g
- ❖ Total Fat: 1g
- ❖ Sat Fat: 0g
- ❖ Protein: 4g
- ❖ Sodium: 278mg

Description Notes:

- This recipe helps to swap red meat that increases the risk of heart disease to bean-based burgers.
- Beans are rich in antioxidants, minerals, vitamins, and dietary fiber. The latter is key for the gut bacteria to thrive and keep us healthy.

Ingredients

- 1 tablespoon ground flaxseed
- 3 tablespoons water
- 1 (14-ounce) can low-sodium kidney beans, drained and rinsed
- 1 small onion, chopped
- ½ cup rolled oats
- 1 teaspoon chili powder

- 1 teaspoon cumin powder
- ½ teaspoon salt
- ½ teaspoon black pepper
- Optional Toppings:
    - Whole grain buns or romaine lettuce leaves (used as wraps)
    - Lettuce, tomato, onion
    - Mustard, ketchup, pickle

Instructions

1. Prepare "flax egg": Combine ground flaxseed and water in a small bowl. Let the mixture sit for 5 minutes to thicken.
2. In a food processor, combine all ingredients and pulse until the mixture is incorporated but still chunky. Alternatively, you can combine ingredients in a bowl and smash with a fork to combine.
3. Allow the mixture to "rest" in the refrigerator for at least 30 minutes.
4. Preheat oven to 400 degrees F. Divide and shape the dough into eight patties. Arrange on a parchment-lined baking sheet.
5. Bake for 8 minutes, flip and bake for another 5-6 minutes until a golden-brown crust forms.
6. Serve immediately. Refrigerate leftovers for up to one week or freeze in an air-tight container for up to 3 months.

Notes:

- Refrigerate leftover patties for up to one week or freeze in an air-tight container for up to 3 months.
- Try this recipe with different beans like white beans or black beans.
- Get creative with different spices and fresh herbs. Try chili powder, cilantro, fresh parsley, garlic powder, or rosemary and thyme.

Chickpea of the Sea Salad

Serves 2

Nutrition Info Per Serving

- ❖ Calories: 439
- ❖ Carbohydrates: 44g
- ❖ Fiber: 14g
- ❖ Total Fat: 25g
- ❖ Sat Fat: 3g
- ❖ Protein: 18g
- ❖ Sodium: 708mg

Description Notes:

- This recipe is a spin on a classic tuna salad.
- Try this easy make-ahead recipe for lunch instead of going to the drive-thru or deli on your lunch break.
- This recipe perfectly combines creamy, crunchy, fresh, and satisfying.

Ingredients

- 1 (14-ounce) can chickpeas, drained and rinsed
- ½ cup celery, chopped
- ½ red onion, chopped'
- 2 tablespoons fresh dill
- 1 lemon
- 3 tablespoons tahini
- 1 teaspoon mustard

- ¼ teaspoon garlic powder
- Salt and pepper to taste
- ¼ cup unsalted sunflower seeds

Instructions

1. Combine all ingredients in a large bowl. Mash with a fork until evenly mixed but still chunky. Alternatively, pulse ingredients in a food processor until combined but still slightly chunky.
2. Serve on bread as a sandwich, with whole grain crackers, or scooped into lettuce boats.

Notes:

- Serve this salad on bread as a sandwich, with whole grain crackers, or scooped into lettuce boats.
- This delicious salad can also be served as a party dip with crackers or cucumber slices.
- The Chickpea of the Sea Salad can be made up to 5 days ahead. Make it on Sunday, and you'll have lunch ready for the whole week.
- For a fun twist, add 2 tablespoons of capers.

Root Vegetable Soup with Citrusy Arugula Salad

Serves 2

Soup Nutrition Info Per Serving

- ❖ Calories: 211
- ❖ Carbohydrates: 45g
- ❖ Fiber: 14g
- ❖ Total Fat: 1g
- ❖ Sat Fat: 0g
- ❖ Protein: 10g
- ❖ Sodium: 345mg

Salad Nutrition Info Per Serving

- ❖ Calories: 122
- ❖ Carbohydrates: 9g
- ❖ Fiber: 5g
- ❖ Total Fat: 9g
- ❖ Sat Fat: 1g
- ❖ Protein: 3g
- ❖ Sodium: 61mg

Description Notes:

- This soup is a gorgeous, vibrant orange!

- It is loaded with beta-carotene (commonly known as Vitamin- A), an antioxidant and an essential vitamin for vision.

- Fresh ginger gives it a warming punch.

- Arugula is healthy for the arteries due to its high nitrate content. It provides a peppery flavor to the dish.

- Kabocha squash is a type of winter squash. It is sweeter than butternut squash.

Soup Ingredients:

- 4 carrots, trimmed and cut into cubes
- 1 kabocha squash, sliced in half and seeds removed
- 1 tablespoon walnut oil (optional)
- ¼ teaspoon salt
- ½ teaspoon black pepper
- 1 yellow onion, diced
- 2 cloves garlic, minced
- 1-inch piece of fresh ginger, peeled
- 4 cups of low-sodium vegetable broth
- ½ cup uncooked red lentils

Salad Ingredients:

- 4 cups arugula
- ¼ cup toasted pepitas (pumpkin seeds)
- 1 serving Mango Citrus Dressing (p. 218)

Instructions:

1. Preheat oven to 400 degrees F. Toss cubed carrots in 2 teaspoons of oil, salt, and pepper. Brush the flesh of the squash with a teaspoon of oil, salt, and pepper. Place carrots

and squash halves (cut side up) on a sheet pan. Bake for 35-40 minutes, until the squash is tender and carrots are golden.

2. Heat a soup pot over medium heat. Add the remaining oil, onion, and garlic. Grate in ginger (if you don't have a grater, finely mince the ginger). Sauté for a few minutes until fragrant. Add the roasted carrots. With a spoon, scoop the tender flesh from the squash. It should separate easily from the skin. Add the squash flesh to the pot. Add the vegetable broth and red lentils and bring to a boil.

3. Reduce to a simmer and cook for 10 minutes until the lentils are tender. Reduce the heat to low, and either blend using an immersion blender or carefully transfer the soup to a blender and blend (work in batches if needed and be very careful blending hot liquids).

4. Toss the arugula and pepitas with the Mango Citrus Dressing for the salad. Serve alongside the soup.

Notes:

- Most hard winter squashes will work for this soup if you can't find kabocha squash. Try acorn or butternut.
- Shortcut: if you don't want to prepare the winter squash, some grocery stores carry frozen cooked winter squash. Toss the frozen squash cubes (about 3 cups) with the carrots and roast to save time.
- To make this meal heartier, top the soup with Everything Bagel Crispy Chickpeas and serve with a slice of whole grain bread spread with avocado.

Red Lentil Curry

Serves 4

Nutrition Info Per Serving

- ❖ Calories: 552
- ❖ Carbohydrates: 98g
- ❖ Fiber: 23g
- ❖ Total Fat: 9g
- ❖ Sat Fat: 7g
- ❖ Protein: 21g
- ❖ Sodium: 441mg

Description Notes:

> This recipe packs a combination of healing properties of the spices, including antioxidant and anti-inflammatory properties found in turmeric, curry powder, cumin, and ginger.

- Red lentils are a great quick-cooking plant protein option.

Ingredients:

- 2 tablespoons avocado oil (optional)
- 1 yellow onion, chopped
- 2 garlic cloves, minced
- 4 medium red potatoes, quartered
- 1 cup cauliflower florets
- 3 cups spinach, roughly chopped
- 1 ½ teaspoons curry powder

- 1 ½ teaspoons ground cumin
- ½ teaspoon ground turmeric
- ½ teaspoon salt
- 1 tablespoon grated fresh ginger
- 1 cup of uncooked red lentils
- 2 cups low-sodium vegetable broth
- 1 (13.66-fluid ounce) can lite coconut milk
- 2 cups brown rice, cooked
- Juice of 1 lime

Instructions:

1. In a large skillet or pot with a lid, sauté onion, garlic, and a pinch of salt over medium heat for 5 minutes or until onion is translucent and fragrant.
2. Add the potatoes, cauliflower, curry powder, cumin, turmeric, and ginger; cook for 5 minutes, stir frequently.
3. Add the broth, coconut milk, lentils, and salt to a simmer. Reduce heat to medium-low, cover with the lid slightly ajar, and cook for 15-20 minutes until lentils and potatoes are tender. Turn off the heat and stir in the spinach.
4. Serve curry over a scoop of brown rice. Top with a squeeze of lime if desired.

Notes:

- Serve this curry with your favorite whole grain. Quinoa, farro, or brown basmati rice all work great.

Sesame Noodle Bowl

Serves 4

Nutrition Info Per Serving

- ❖ Calories: 353
- ❖ Carbohydrates: 59g
- ❖ Fiber: 7g
- ❖ Total Fat: 7g
- ❖ Sat Fat: 1g
- ❖ Protein: 21g
- ❖ Sodium: 976mg

Description Notes:

- This can be enjoyed warm or cold, fresh or made ahead.

Ingredients:

- 1 (8-ounce) package of buckwheat soba noodles
- 2 teaspoons avocado oil (optional)
- 2 cups broccoli florets
- 1 red bell pepper, seeded and sliced
- 1 cup snow peas
- 1 cup edamame beans
- ¼ cup green onion
- 2 tablespoons tamari/low-sodium soy sauce
- 1 tablespoon grated fresh ginger

- 2 cloves garlic, minced
- 2 tablespoons toasted sesame seeds

Instructions:

1. Cook noodles according to package directions.
2. Heat skillet over medium-high heat. Add optional oil, broccoli, bell pepper, snow peas, edamame, and green onions. Sauté just until vegetables are tender. Turn off the heat, and add tamari, ginger, garlic, and toasted sesame seeds. Toss to coat.
3. Divide noodles into two bowls and top with vegetables.

Notes:

- To make this meal extra veggie-packed, swap the soba noodles for "noodles" made from spiralized zucchini or sweet potatoes.
- Enjoy this dish warm or cold (it makes excellent leftovers for lunch).

Slow Cooker Tuscan White Bean Stew

Serves 4

Nutrition Info Per Serving

- ❖ Calories: 431
- ❖ Carbohydrates: 89g
- ❖ Fiber: 28g
- ❖ Total Fat: 1g
- ❖ Sat Fat: 0g
- ❖ Protein: 22g
- ❖ Sodium: 941mg

Description Notes:

- A slow cooker can be an option to manage cooking time when juggling daily routines.

- This warm, hearty meal is brightened with a squeeze of lemon and fresh kale.

- Don't own a slow cooker? Make this recipe on the stovetop using a large soup pot. Combine all ingredients, and simmer until the vegetables are tender (about 30 minutes).

Ingredients:

- 1 yellow onion, diced
- 3 cloves garlic, peeled and minced
- 6 carrots, chopped
- 6 ribs of celery, chopped
- 2 large or 4 small yukon gold potatoes, cut into ½-inch cubes

- 2 (15-ounce) cans low-sodium cannellini beans
- 6 cups low-sodium vegetable broth
- 1 teaspoon salt
- 2 tablespoon salt-free Italian seasoning blend
- 2 cups fresh kale, chopped
- Juice of 1 lemon

Instructions:

1. In a slow cooker, combine all ingredients except kale and lemon juice. Set the slow cooker on high and cook for 4 to 5 hours. Alternatively, set the slow cooker on the lowest setting and cook for 8 to 10 hours.
2. Just before serving, stir in the fresh kale and lemon juice. Top with Plant-based Parmesan (p. 227) and serve with crusty whole-grain bread or crackers.

Notes:

- Try this recipe with different types of vegetables or beans. Swap the kale for spinach, add shiitake mushrooms, or try it with chickpeas or lima beans instead of cannellini beans.

Ultimate Chopped Salad

Serves 1

Nutrition Info Per Serving

- ❖ Calories: 413
- ❖ Carbohydrates: 65g
- ❖ Fiber: 16g
- ❖ Total Fat: 13g
- ❖ Sat Fat: 2g
- ❖ Protein: 16g
- ❖ Sodium: 214mg

Description Notes:

- This recipe helps someone see that 1) making a salad at home doesn't need to be intimidating, and 2) salad can make a very filling meal!
- Anything goes with this one - the cook can get creative with whatever veggies and dressings they love and have available.

Ingredients:

- ½ cup quinoa, cooked
- ½ cup chickpeas, drained and rinsed
- 2 cups romaine or green leaf lettuce, chopped
- ½ cup corn kernels, thawed from frozen or sliced of the cob
- ½ cup cucumber, chopped
- ½ cup cherry tomatoes

- ¼ avocado
- 1 serving Herby Ranch Dressing (p. 209)

Instructions:

1. Combine all ingredients in a large bowl and toss with dressing. Enjoy immediately.

Notes:

- The Ultimate Chopped Salad is the "no rules" meal! Try different combinations of whole grains, beans, veggies, and dressings you love.

Tofu Poke Bowl

Serves 4

Nutrition Info Per Serving

- ❖ Calories: 313
- ❖ Carbohydrates: 33g
- ❖ Fiber: 7g
- ❖ Total Fat: 14g
- ❖ Sat Fat: 2g
- ❖ Protein:15g
- ❖ Sodium: 766mg

Description Notes:

- This recipe swaps protein for healthy, anti-cancer tofu options from the high-mercury load fish such as tuna traditionally used in poke bowls.

Ingredients:

- 2 cups brown rice, cooked
- 1 14-ounce block of firm tofu
- ⅓ cup tamari/low-sodium soy sauce
- 2 teaspoons toasted sesame oil (optional)
- 1 tablespoon rice vinegar
- 1 clove garlic
- ⅛ teaspoon powdered ginger
- 1 tablespoon toasted sesame seeds
- ½ cucumber, sliced

- 4 red radishes, sliced
- ¼ cup green onion, chopped
- 1 avocado, cut into slices
- Optional for serving: sriracha, pickled ginger, lime wedge

Instructions:

1. Prepare the tofu:
    a. Drain liquid from the tofu and press the block between two layers of paper towels to remove some of the moisture.
    b. Cut the pressed tofu block into ½ inch cubes.
    c. Whisk together tamari, sesame oil, rice vinegar, garlic, ginger, and toasted sesame seeds in a shallow dish. Add cubed tofu and toss to coat. Marinate for 30 minutes.
2. Assemble poke bowls: divide rice and marinated tofu among 4 bowls. Top with sliced cucumber, radish, green onion, and avocado. Add additional optional toppings and enjoy!

Notes:

- Short on time? Use edamame beans instead of the tofu and whisk the marinade into a sauce to pour over your bowl.
- Set up a build-your-own Poke Bowl bar for your family or dinner guests.

SNACKS + DESSERTS

One Bowl Oatmeal Cookies

Makes 12 Cookies

Nutrition Info Per Serving

- ❖ Calories: 76
- ❖ Carbohydrates: 10g
- ❖ Fiber: 2g
- ❖ Total Fat: 3g
- ❖ Sat Fat: 0g
- ❖ Protein: 2g
- ❖ Sodium: 23g

Description Notes:

- Cookies that are delicious enough for dessert but healthy enough to be a snack too
- The nut butter and banana make healthy substitutes for butter and eggs, respectively.

Ingredients:

- 1 cup old-fashioned oats
- 2 ripe banana
- ¼ cup almond butter
- ½ teaspoon vanilla extract
- ½ teaspoon baking powder
- Pinch of salt
- Optional mix-ins: dairy-free chocolate chips, dried cranberries, raisins, pecans, pumpkin seeds

Instructions:

1. Preheat oven to 350 degrees F.
2. Mash banana and nut butter together in a bowl until it forms a smooth paste.
3. Add remaining ingredients and mix until incorporated.
4. Scoop heaping tablespoon-sized balls of dough onto a parchment paper-lined cookie sheet.
5. Bake for 12-15 minutes. Let cool before enjoying.

Stuffed Dates

Serves 1 person (2 dates)

Nutrition Info Per Serving

- Calories: 234
- Carbohydrates: 17g
- Fiber: 3g
- Total Fat: 16g
- Sat Fat: 3g
- Protein: 8g
- Sodium: 138

Nutrition info is for two dates, 2 tablespoons peanut butter, and ½ teaspoon cinnamon.

Description Notes:

- Dates make the perfect whole-food sweet treat. It has a distinct sweet flavor and, when ripe, has a chewy consistency.

Ingredients:

- 2 Medjool dates
- Filling options:
    - 2 tablespoons peanut butter, almond butter, or any nut or seed butter
    - 2 walnut halves
    - 2 tablespoons almond ricotta or other dairy-free soft 'cheese'
- Topping options (quantities given per date):

- 2 teaspoons shredded coconut
- 1 teaspoon cacao nibs
- 2 teaspoon dairy-free chocolate chips
- ½ teaspoon cinnamon
- 2 teaspoon hemp seeds
- 2 teaspoons chopped nuts

Instructions:

1. Carefully slice down one side of each date, keeping the other side intact (so it opens like a book). Remove pits.
2. Place a dollop of your filling of choice inside each date. Sprinkle with toppings. Gently press the back together without closing the date all the way (serve like a half-open book).
3. Combination ideas:
    a. Peanut butter + cacao nibs
    b. Almond ricotta + shredded coconut + chocolate chips
    c. Tahini + cinnamon

Garlicky Edamame Dip

Yields about 2 ½ cups or about 6 ¼-cup servings

Nutrition Info Per Serving

- Calories: 125
- Carbohydrates: 8g
- Fiber: 3g
- Total Fat: 8g
- Sat Fat: 1g
- Protein: 7g
- Sodium: 39mg

Description Notes:

- Tahini is a sesame seed paste and is a good source of calcium.
- Use it as a sandwich spread or dip.

INGREDIENTS

- 2 cups frozen edamame beans, thawed
- ¼ cup tahini
- Juice of 1 lemon
- 2 garlic cloves
- ½ teaspoons paprika
- Salt to taste
- ¼ - ½ cup water, adjust to preferred consistency

INSTRUCTIONS

1. Add all ingredients except water to a food processor or blender. Blend until smooth.

2. While the food processor runs, add water - a tablespoon at a time - until the bean dip reaches your preferred consistency.

3. Store in an air-tight container in the refrigerator for up to a week.

Notes:

- Serve this dip with sliced veggies for dipping. Try bell peppers, radishes, carrot sticks, celery, or even room-temperature roasted vegetables cauliflower florets.

- For a more filling snack, serve with whole grain crackers.

- This savory, protein-packed dip makes an excellent sandwich or wrap spread.

Cacao Mousse with Fresh Berries

Serves 4

Nutrition Info Per Serving

- ❖ Calories: 145
- ❖ Carbohydrates: 29g
- ❖ Fiber: 7g
- ❖ Total Fat: 5g
- ❖ Sat Fat: 1g
- ❖ Protein: 2g
- ❖ Sodium: 14g

Description Notes:

- A very creamy, rich, decadent dessert!
- Cacao powder is a rich source of antioxidants.
- Using tofu adds healthy protein to make a dessert and replaces butter, heavy cream, etc.

Ingredients:

- ½ avocado
- 1 12-ounce package of silken tofu
- ½ cup pitted Medjool dates
- ¼ cup cacao powder
- ½ teaspoon vanilla extract
- ¼ teaspoon cinnamon
- Pinch of salt

- Pinch of cayenne (optional)
- 2 cups fresh berries

Instructions:

1. Soak dates in a bowl of water for at least 4 hours. Drain.
2. Combine the avocado, silken tofu, soaked dates, cacao powder, vanilla extract, cinnamon, salt, and optional cayenne in a food processor or blender. Blend until completely smooth. Chill in the refrigerator for at least 30 min.
3. When ready to serve, scoop into bowls and top with fresh berries.

Notes:

- Serve this luscious dessert with any fruit that is in season. Pomegranate seeds, banana slices, and cherries are all perfect pairings.

Everything Bagel Crispy Chickpeas

Serves 4

Nutrition Info Per Serving

- Calories: 123
- Carbohydrates: 20g
- Fiber: 6g
- Total Fat: 2g
- Sat Fat: 0g
- Protein: 7g
- Sodium: 415mg

Description Notes:

- Makes a perfect crunchy, salty snack.
- Making these at home minimizes consuming excess oil, sugar, and salt that invariably comes with buying them packaged.

Ingredients:

- 1 (15-ounce) can chickpeas
- 1 tablespoon walnut oil (optional)
- 1 teaspoon dried onion
- 1 teaspoon onion powder
- 1 teaspoon dried garlic
- 1 teaspoon garlic powder
- 1 teaspoon sesame seeds
- 1 teaspoon poppy seeds

- ½ teaspoon coarse salt

Instructions:

1. Drain chickpeas. If you are planning to use oil, rinse chickpeas with water. If you are omitting oil, do not rinse. Then, spread out on a towel to dry completely for at least 30 minutes.

2. Preheat oven to 350 degrees F. When chickpeas are dry, toss with oil (optional). Spread in a single layer on a baking sheet. Bake for 45 minutes until chickpeas are golden brown and fairly crisp.

3. While chickpeas bake, combine the remaining ingredients in a medium bowl.

4. As soon as the chickpeas are done baking, remove from the oven and toss in the seasoning mix. Spread chickpeas in an even layer on the baking sheet and let cool before serving.

Cheesy Kale Chips

Serves 2

Nutrition Info Per Serving

- ❖ Calories: 51
- ❖ Carbohydrates: 6g
- ❖ Fiber: 5g
- ❖ Total Fat: 1g
- ❖ Sat Fat: 0g
- ❖ Protein: 6g
- ❖ Sodium: 325mg

Description Notes:

- An unexpected crispy, salty snack and an excellent way to add in more leafy greens
- Kid-friendly

Ingredients:

- 1 bunch of kale
- ½ tablespoon walnut oil (optional)
- ¼ teaspoons salt
- 2 tablespoons nutritional yeast

Instructions:

1. Strip kale leaves off of the stems and tear leaves into chip-sized pieces. Rinse and let dry completely.

2. Preheat oven to 300 degrees F. Massage dry kale leaves with oil (optional) and toss with salt and nutritional yeast to coat.
3. Spread leaves in a single layer on a baking sheet without overlapping any of the leaves (this is very important!).
4. Bake for 15 minutes but watch them closely - they will burn easily! Remove from the oven and cool on the baking sheet for about 5 minutes.

Notes:

- Try different seasoning combinations:
    - Massage dry kale leaves with BBQ sauce before baking
    - Add garlic powder and onion powder for a Ranch flavor

Seasonal Fruit Crumble

Serves 6

Nutrition Info Per Serving

- ❖ Calories: 160
- ❖ Carbohydrates: 29g
- ❖ Fiber: 4g
- ❖ Total Fat: 5g
- ❖ Sat Fat: 0g
- ❖ Protein: 2g
- ❖ Sodium: 51mg

Description Notes:

- A nourishing dessert recipe that adapts to the seasons

Ingredients:

- ¾ cup old-fashioned oats
- ¼ cup chopped nuts (pecans, walnuts, almonds, etc.)
- ½ teaspoon cinnamon
- ⅛ teaspoon salt
- 1 tablespoon walnut oil (optional)
- ¼ cup maple syrup or date syrup divided
- 4 cups chopped/sliced fruit (fresh berries, apples, pears, peaches, plums, etc.)
- Juice of ½ lemon

Instructions:

1. Preheat oven to 400 degrees F.

2. Add the oats, nuts, cinnamon, salt, optional walnut oil, and 2 tablespoons of maple or date syrup in a medium bowl. Stir until combined. Set aside.

3. Add the chopped/sliced fruit, half of the maple syrup, and the lemon juice in a pie pan or casserole dish. Stir until combined, then spread into an even layer in the dish.

4. Sprinkle the oat mixture evenly over the fruit. Bake for 20 minutes until the crumble topping is browned and the fruit filling is bubbling.

REFERENCES

CHAPTER 1. WITHERING ALLIANCE: EXCESS BODY WEIGHT

[1] Laron, Z. (2015). Lessons from 50 Years of Study of Laron Syndrome. *Endocrine Practice,* 21(12), 1395–1402. https://doi.org/10.4158/ep15939.ra

[2] Fürstenberger, G., & Senn, H. (2002). Insulin-like growth factors and cancer. *Lancet Oncology, 3*(5), 298–302. https://doi.org/10.1016/s1470-2045(02)00731-3

[3] Cox, T. O., Lundgren, P., Nath, K., & Thaiss, C. A. (2022). Metabolic control by the microbiome. *Genome Medicine,* 14(1). https://doi.org/10.1186/s13073-022-01092-0

[4] The Integrative Human Microbiome Project: Dynamic Analysis of Microbiome-Host Omics Profiles during Periods of Human Health and Disease. (2014). *Cell Host & Microbe,* 16(3), 276–289. https://doi.org/10.1016/j.chom.2014.08.014

[5] Qin, J., Li, R., Raes, J., Arumugam, M., Burgdorf, K. S., Manichanh, C., . . . Wang, J. (2010). A human gut microbial gene catalogue established by metagenomic sequencing. *Nature,* 464(7285), 59–65. https://doi.org/10.1038/nature08821

[6] Wikipedia contributors. (2023, December 17). Ramayana. Retrieved from https://en.wikipedia.org/wiki/Ramayana

[7] Wig, N. N. (2004). Hanuman complex and its resolution: an illustration of psychotherapy from Indian mythology. *Indian Journal of Psychiatry,* 46(1), 25-28.

[8] Glanz, K., Bader, M., & Iyer, S. (2012). Retail grocery store marketing strategies and obesity. *American Journal of Preventive Medicine,* 42(5), 503–512. https://doi.org/10.1016/j.amepre.2012.01.013

[9] Moss, M. (2013). Salt, sugar, fat: How the Food Giants Hooked Us. Random House.

[10] Coll, A. P., Farooqi, I. S., & O'Rahilly, S. (2007). The hormonal control of food intake. *Cell,* 129(2), 251–262. https://doi.org/10.1016/j.cell.2007.04.001

[11] Yeung, A. Y., Tady, P. (2023, January 3). Physiology, obesity neurohormonal appetite and satiety control. *StatPearls.* StatPearls Publishing. Retrieved from https://www.ncbi.nlm.nih.gov/books/NBK555906/

[12] Klok, M. D., Jakobsdottir, S., & Drent, M. L. (2006). The role of leptin and ghrelin in the regulation of food intake and body weight in humans: a review. *Obesity Reviews,* 8(1), 21–34. https://doi.org/10.1111/j.1467-789x.2006.00270.x

[13] Liu, J., Yang, X., Yu, S., & Zheng, R. (2018). The leptin resistance. *Advances in Experimental Medicine and Biology* (pp. 145–163). https://doi.org/10.1007/978-981-13-1286-1_8

[14] Engin, A. B. (2017). Diet-Induced obesity and the mechanism of leptin resistance. *Advances in Experimental Medicine and Biology* (pp. 381–397). https://doi.org/10.1007/978-3-319-48382-5_16

[15] Sáinz, N., Barrenetxe, J., Moreno-Aliaga, M. J., & Martínéz, J. A. (2015). Leptin resistance and diet-induced obesity: central and peripheral actions of leptin. *Metabolism,* 64(1), 35–46. https://doi.org/10.1016/j.metabol.2014.10.015

[16] Vancamelbeke, M., & Vermeire, S. (2017). The intestinal barrier: a fundamental role in health and disease. *Expert Review of Gastroenterology & Hepatology,* 11(9), 821–834. https://doi.org/10.1080/17474124.2017.1343143

[17] Banks, W. A., Farr, S. A., Salameh, T. S., Niehoff, M. L., Rhea, E. M., Morley, J. E., . . . Craft, S. (2017). Triglycerides cross the blood–brain barrier and induce central leptin and insulin receptor resistance. *International Journal of Obesity,* 42(3), 391–397. https://doi.org/10.1038/ijo.2017.231 .

[18] Turner, J. R. (2017). The mucosal barrier at a glance. *Journal of Cell Science.* https://doi.org/10.1242/jcs.193482

[19] Usuda, H., Okamoto, T., & Wada, K. (2021). Leaky gut: Effect of dietary fiber and fats on microbiome and intestinal barrier. *International Journal of Molecular Sciences,* 22(14), 7613. https://doi.org/10.3390/ijms22147613

[20] Camilleri, M. (2019). Leaky gut: mechanisms, measurement and clinical implications in humans. *Gut,* 68(8), 1516–1526. https://doi.org/10.1136/gutjnl-2019-318427

[21] Hailman, E., Lichenstein, H. S., Wurfel, M. M., Miller, D. S., Johnson, D. A., Kelley, M. J., . . . Wright, S. D. (1994). Lipopolysaccharide (LPS)-binding protein accelerates the binding of LPS to CD14. *Journal of Experimental Medicine*, 179(1), 269–277. https://doi.org/10.1084/jem.179.1.269

[22] Chelakkot, C., Ghim, J., & Ryu, S. H. (2018). Mechanisms regulating intestinal barrier integrity and its pathological implications. *Experimental & Molecular Medicine*, 50(8), 1–9. https://doi.org/10.1038/s12276-018-0126-x

[23] Erlanson-Albertsson, C., & Stenkula, K. G. (2021). The importance of food for endotoxemia and an inflammatory response. *International Journal of Molecular Sciences*, 22(17), 9562. https://doi.org/10.3390/ijms22179562

[24] Fuke, N., Nagata, N., Suganuma, H., & Ota, T. (2019). Regulation of Gut Microbiota and Metabolic Endotoxemia with Dietary Factors. *Nutrients*, 11(10), 2277. https://doi.org/10.3390/nu11102277

[25] Gwak, M., & Chang, S. (2021). Gut-Brain connection: microbiome, gut barrier, and environmental sensors. *Immune Network*, 21(3). https://doi.org/10.4110/in.2021.21.e20

[26] Little, T. J., Horowitz, M., & Feinle-Bisset, C. (2005). Role of cholecystokinin in appetite control and body weight regulation. *Obesity Reviews*, 6(4), 297–306. https://doi.org/10.1111/j.1467-789x.2005.00212.x

[27] Overby, H., & Ferguson, J. F. (2021). Gut Microbiota-Derived Short-Chain Fatty Acids Facilitate Microbiota:Host Cross talk and

Modulate Obesity and Hypertension. *Current Hypertension Reports*, 23(2). https://doi.org/10.1007/s11906-020-01125-2

[28]Fusco, W. G., Bernabeu, M., Cintoni, M., Porcari, S., Rinninella, E., Kaitsas, F., . . . Ianiro, G. (2023). Short-Chain Fatty-Acid-Producing bacteria: key components of the human gut microbiota. *Nutrients, 15*(9), 2211. https://doi.org/10.3390/nu15092211

[29] Dalile, B., Van Oudenhove, L., Vervliet, B., & Verbeke, K. (2019). The role of short-chain fatty acids in microbiota–gut–brain communication. *Nature Reviews Gastroenterology & Hepatology,* 16(8), 461–478. https://doi.org/10.1038/s41575-019-0157-3

[30]Carabotti, M. (2015, June 1). The gut-brain axis: interactions between enteric microbiota, central and enteric nervous systems. *Annals of gastroenterology, 28*(2), 203–209. Retrieved from https://www.ncbi.nlm.nih.gov/pmc/articles/PMC4367209/

[31]Kadyan, S., Sharma, A., Arjmandi, B. H., Singh, P., & Nagpal, R. (2022). Prebiotic potential of dietary beans and pulses and their resistant starch for Aging-Associated gut and metabolic health. *Nutrients,* 14(9), 1726. https://doi.org/10.3390/nu14091726

[32]Singh, B., Singh, J., Shevkani, K., Singh, N., & Kaur, A. (2016). Bioactive constituents in pulses and their health benefits. *Journal of Food Science and Technology,* 54(4), 858–870. https://doi.org/10.1007/s13197-016-2391-9

[33]Loarca-Piña, G., García-Gasca, T., Guevara-González, R. G., Ramos-Gómez, M., & Oomah, B. D. (2012). Human Gut Flora-Fermented Nondigestible Fraction from Cooked Bean (Phaseolus vulgaris L.) Modifies Protein Expression Associated with Apoptosis, Cell Cycle Arrest, and Proliferation in Human Adenocarcinoma Colon Cancer Cells. *Journal of Agricultural and Food Chemistry,* 60(51), 12443–12450. https://doi.org/10.1021/jf303940r

[34] De Angelis, M., Ferrocino, I., Calabrese, F. M., De Filippis, F., Cavallo, N., Siragusa, S., . . . Cocolin, L. S. (2020). Diet influences the functions of the human intestinal microbiome. *Scientific Reports*, *10*(1). https://doi.org/10.1038/s41598-020-61192-y

[35] Krajmalnik-Brown, R., Ilhan, Z. E., Kang, D. W., & DiBaise, J. K. (2012). Effects of gut microbes on nutrient absorption and energy regulation. *Nutrition in Clinical Practice*, 27(2), 201–214. https://doi.org/10.1177/0884533611436116

[36] Di Costanzo, M., De Paulis, N., & Biasucci, G. (2021). Butyrate: A Link between Early Life Nutrition and Gut Microbiome in the Development of Food Allergy. *Life*, 11(5), 384. https://doi.org/10.3390/life11050384

[37] Chao, A. M., Grilo, C. M., White, M. A., & Sinha, R. (2015). Food cravings mediate the relationship between chronic stress and body mass index. *Journal of Health Psychology*, 20(6), 721–729. https://doi.org/10.1177/1359105315573448

[38] Chao, A. M., Jastreboff, A. M., White, M. A., Grilo, C. M., & Sinha, R. (2017). Stress, cortisol, and other appetite-related hormones: Prospective prediction of 6-month changes in food cravings and weight. *Obesity*, *25*(4), 713–720. https://doi.org/10.1002/oby.21790

[39] Kuckuck, S., Van Der Valk, E. S., Scheurink, A., Van Der Voorn, B., Iyer, A. M., Visser, J. A., . . . Van Der Valk, E. S. (2022). Glucocorticoids, stress and eating: The mediating role of appetite-regulating hormones. *Obesity Reviews*, 24(3). https://doi.org/10.1111/obr.13539

[40] Moeller, S. J., Couto, L., Cohen, V., Lalazar, Y., Makotkine, I., Williams, N., . . . Geer, E. B. (2016). Glucocorticoid Regulation of Food-Choice Behavior in Humans: Evidence from Cushing's Syndrome. *Frontiers in Neuroscience*, 10. https://doi.org/10.3389/fnins.2016.00021

[41] Wallace, C. W., & Fordahl, S. C. (2021). Obesity and dietary fat influence dopamine neurotransmission: exploring the convergence of metabolic state, physiological stress, and inflammation on dopaminergic control of food intake. *Nutrition Research Reviews*, 35(2), 236–251. https://doi.org/10.1017/s0954422421000196

[42] Thanarajah, S. E., DiFeliceantonio, A. G., Albus, K., Kuzmanovic, B., Rigoux, L., Iglesias, S., . . . Small, D. M. (2023). Habitual daily intake of a sweet and fatty snack modulates reward processing in humans. *Cell Metabolism*, 35(4), 571-584.e6. https://doi.org/10.1016/j.cmet.2023.02.015

[43] Fontana, L., Eagon, J. C., Trujillo, M. E., Scherer, P. E., & Klein, S. (2007). Visceral fat adipokine secretion is associated with systemic inflammation in obese humans. *Diabetes*, 56(4), 1010–1013. https://doi.org/10.2337/db06-1656

[44] Mukherjee, S., Skrede, S., Haugstøyl, M. E., López, M., & Fernø, J. (2023). Peripheral and central macrophages in obesity. *Frontiers in Endocrinology*, 14. https://doi.org/10.3389/fendo.2023.1232171

[45] Obara-Michlewska, M. (2022). The contribution of astrocytes to obesity-associated metabolic disturbances. *Journal of Nanjing Medical University*, 36(5), 299. https://doi.org/10.7555/jbr.36.20200020

[46] Makki, K., Deehan, E. C., Walter, J., & Bäckhed, F. (2018). The impact of dietary fiber on gut microbiota in host health and disease. *Cell Host & Microbe*, 23(6), 705–715. https://doi.org/10.1016/j.chom.2018.05.012

[47] Ellulu, M. S., Patimah, I., Khaza'ai, H., Rahmat, A., & Abed, Y. (2017). Obesity and inflammation: the linking mechanism and the complications. *Archives of Medical Science*, 4, 851–863. https://doi.org/10.5114/aoms.2016.58928

[48]Lisle, D. J., & Goldhamer, A. (2007). The pleasure trap: Mastering the Force that Undermines Health & Happiness. Book Publishing Company.
[49]Vinolo, M. a. R., Rodrigues, H. G., Nachbar, R. T., & Curi, R. (2011). Regulation of inflammation by short chain fatty acids. *Nutrients*, 3(10), 858–876. https://doi.org/10.3390/nu3100858
[50] Breast cancer facts & figures. (n.d.). Retrieved from https://www.cancer.org/research/cancer-facts-statistics/breast-cancer-facts-figures.html

CHAPTER 2. TERROR WITH AN ACHILLES HEEL: CANCER

[51] Angelina Jolie. (2013, May 14). Retrieved from https://www.nytimes.com/2013/05/14/opinion/my-medical-choice.html
[52] Yoshida, K., & Miki, Y. (2004). Role of BRCA1 and BRCA2 as regulators of DNA repair, transcription, and cell cycle in response to DNA damage. *Cancer Science*, 95(11), 866–871. https://doi.org/10.1111/j.1349-7006.2004.tb02195.x
[53]Saha, S. K., Lee, S. B., Won, J., Choi, H. Y., Kim, K., Yang, G., . . . Cho, S. (2017). Correlation between Oxidative Stress, Nutrition, and Cancer Initiation. *International Journal of Molecular Sciences*, 18(7), 1544. https://doi.org/10.3390/ijms18071544
[54]Ames, B. N. (1983). Dietary carcinogens and anticarcinogens. *Science*, 221(4617), 1256–1264. https://doi.org/10.1126/science.6351251
[55]Di Meo, S., & Venditti, P. (2020). Evolution of the knowledge of free radicals and other oxidants. *Oxidative Medicine and Cellular Longevity*, 2020, 1–32. https://doi.org/10.1155/2020/9829176
[56]Litwinienko, G., & Ingold, K. U. (2004). Abnormal solvent effects on hydrogen atom abstraction. 2. Resolution of the curcumin antioxidant controversy. The role of sequential proton loss

electron transfer. *The Journal of Organic Chemistry,* 69(18), 5888–5896. https://doi.org/10.1021/jo049254j

[57]Oyagbemi, A. A., Azeez, O. I., & Saba, A. B. (2009). Interactions between reactive oxygen species and cancer: the roles of natural dietary antioxidants and their molecular mechanisms of action. *Asian Pacific journal of cancer prevention : APJCP,* 10(4), 535–544. Retrieved from https://pubmed.ncbi.nlm.nih.gov/19827865

[58]Merlin, J. P. J., Rupasinghe, H. V., Dellaire, G., & Murphy, K. (2021). Role of dietary Antioxidants in P53-Mediated Cancer Chemoprevention and Tumor Suppression. *Oxidative Medicine and Cellular Longevity,* 2021, 1–18. https://doi.org/10.1155/2021/9924328

[59] Tapsell, L. C., Hemphill, I., Cobiac, L., Patch, C. S., Sullivan, D., Fenech, M., . . . Inge, K. E. (2006). Health benefits of herbs and spices: the past, the present, the future. *Medical Journal of Australia,* 185(S4). https://doi.org/10.5694/j.1326-5377.2006.tb00548.x

[60]Chatterjee, N., & Walker, G. C. (2017). Mechanisms of DNA damage, repair, and mutagenesis. *Environmental and Molecular Mutagenesis,* 58(5), 235–263. https://doi.org/10.1002/em.22087

[61] Mader, S. S. (1996b). *Biology.*

[62] Cox, G. W. (1997). *Conservation Biology: Concepts and Applications.* McGraw-Hill Science, Engineering & Mathematics.

[63] Hawkins, I. W. (2018). *Promoting biodiversity in food systems.* CRC Press eBooks. https://doi.org/10.1201/b22084

[64]Clinton, S. K., Truex, C. R., Imrey, P. B., & Visek, W. J. (1980). DIETARY PROTEIN AND MIXED FUNCTION OXIDASE ACTIVITY. Elsevier eBooks (pp. 1129–1132). https://doi.org/10.1016/b978-0-12-187702-6.50096-7

[65]Nebert, D. W., & Dalton, T. P. (2006). The role of cytochrome P450 enzymes in endogenous signalling pathways and environmental carcinogenesis. *Nature Reviews Cancer,* 6(12), 947–960. https://doi.org/10.1038/nrc2015

[66] Ld, Y., & Tc, C. (1992). The sustained development of preneoplastic lesions depends on high protein intake. *Nutrition and Cancer*, 18(2), 131–142. https://doi.org/10.1080/01635589209514213

[67] Callaway, E. (2015). How elephants avoid cancer. *Nature.* https://doi.org/10.1038/nature.2015.18534

[68] Padariya, M., Jooste, M., Hupp, T. R., Fåhræus, R., Vojtesek, B., Vollrath, F., . . . Karakostis, K. (2022). The Elephant Evolved p53 Isoforms that Escape MDM2-Mediated Repression and Cancer. *Molecular Biology and Evolution*, 39(7). https://doi.org/10.1093/molbev/msac149

[69] Park, J. Y., Mitrou, P., Keen, J., Dahm, C. C., Luben, R., McTaggart, A., . . . Rodwell, S. A. (2010). Lifestyle factors and p53 mutation patterns in colorectal cancer patients in the EPIC-Norfolk study. *Mutagenesis*, 25(4), 351–358. https://doi.org/10.1093/mutage/geq012

[70] Merlin, J. P. J., Rupasinghe, H. V., Dellaire, G., & Murphy, K. (2021b). Role of dietary Antioxidants in P53-Mediated Cancer Chemoprevention and Tumor Suppression. *Oxidative Medicine and Cellular Longevity*, 2021, 1–18. https://doi.org/10.1155/2021/9924328

[71] Grimberg, A. (2003b). Mechanisms by which IGF-I May Promote Cancer. *Cancer Biology & Therapy*, 2(6), 628–633. https://doi.org/10.4161/cbt.2.6.678

[72] Crowe, F. L., Key, T. J., Allen, N. E., Appleby, P. N., Roddam, A., Overvad, K., . . . Kaaks, R. (2009). The Association between Diet and Serum Concentrations of IGF-I, IGFBP-1, IGFBP-2, and IGFBP-3 in the European Prospective Investigation into Cancer and Nutrition. *Cancer Epidemiology, Biomarkers & Prevention*, 18(5), 1333–1340. https://doi.org/10.1158/1055-9965.epi-08-0781

[73] Levine, M. E., Suárez, J., Brandhorst, S., Balasubramanian, P., Cheng, C., Madia, F., . . . Longo, V. D. (2014). Low Protein Intake Is Associated with a Major Reduction in IGF-1, Cancer, and

Overall Mortality in the 65 and Younger but Not Older Population. *Cell Metabolism,* 19(3), 407–417. https://doi.org/10.1016/j.cmet.2014.02.006

[74] WCRF International. (2022, April 14). Diet, activity and cancer - WCRF International. Retrieved from https://wcrf.org/diet-activity-and-cancer/

[75] Ml, M., & Chiarelli, F. (2013). Obesity and Growth during Childhood and Puberty. In World review of nutrition and dietetics (pp. 135–141). https://doi.org/10.1159/000342545

[76] Cheng, G., Buyken, A. E., Shi, L., Karaolis-Danckert, N., Kroke, A., Wudy, S. A., . . . Remer, T. (2012). Beyond overweight: nutrition as an important lifestyle factor influencing timing of puberty. *Nutrition Reviews,* 70(3), 133–152. https://doi.org/10.1111/j.1753-4887.2011.00461.x

[77] Laron, Z., Kauli, R., Lapkina, L., & Werner, H. (2017). IGF-I deficiency, longevity and cancer protection of patients with Laron syndrome. *Mutation Research/Reviews in Mutation Research*, 772, 123–133. https://doi.org/10.1016/j.mrrev.2016.08.002

[78] Janecka, A., Kołodziej-Rzepa, M., & Biesaga, B. (2016). Clinical and Molecular Features of Laron Syndrome, A Genetic Disorder Protecting from Cancer. *In vivo (Athens, Greece)*, 30(4), 375–381. Retrieved from https://pubmed.ncbi.nlm.nih.gov/27381597

[79] Snowdon, D. A. (1988). Animal product consumption and mortality because of all causes combined, coronary heart disease, stroke, diabetes, and cancer in Seventh-day Adventists. *The American Journal of Clinical Nutrition*, 48(3), 739–748. https://doi.org/10.1093/ajcn/48.3.739

[80] Orlich, M. J., Mashchak, A., Jaceldo-Siegl, K., Utt, J., Knutsen, S. F., Sveen, L. E., & Fraser, G. E. (2022). Dairy foods, calcium intakes, and risk of incident prostate cancer in Adventist Health Study–2. *The American Journal of Clinical Nutrition*, 116(2), 314–324. https://doi.org/10.1093/ajcn/nqac093

[81] Segovia-Siapco, G., & Sabaté, J. (2018). Health and sustainability outcomes of vegetarian dietary patterns: a revisit of the EPIC-Oxford and the Adventist Health Study-2 cohorts. *European Journal of Clinical Nutrition*, 72(S1), 60–70. https://doi.org/10.1038/s41430-018-0310-z

[82] Sutter, D., & Bender, N. (2021). Nutrient status and growth in vegan children. *Nutrition Research*, 91, 13–25. https://doi.org/10.1016/j.nutres.2021.04.005

[83] Key, T. J., Appleby, P. N., Barnes, I., Reeves, G., & Hormones, E. (2002). Endogenous sex hormones and breast cancer in Postmenopausal Women: Reanalysis of nine prospective studies. *JNCI: Journal of the National Cancer Institute*, 94(8), 606–616. https://doi.org/10.1093/jnci/94.8.606

[84] Huang, M., Liu, J., Lin, X., Goto, A., Song, Y., Tinker, L. F., . . . Liu, S. (2017). Relationship between dietary carbohydrates intake and circulating sex hormone-binding globulin levels in postmenopausal women. *Journal of Diabetes*, 10(6), 467–477. https://doi.org/10.1111/1753-0407.12550

[85] Wayne, S. J., Neuhouser, M. L., Ulrich, C. M., Koprowski, C., Baumgartner, K. B., Baumgartner, R. N., . . . Ballard-Barbash, R. (2007). Dietary fiber is associated with serum sex hormones and insulin-related peptides in postmenopausal breast cancer survivors. *Breast Cancer Research and Treatment*, 112(1), 149–158. https://doi.org/10.1007/s10549-007-9834-y

[86] Goldin, B. R., Adlercreutz, H., Gorbach, S. L., Warram, J. H., Dwyer, J., Swenson, L., & Woods, M. N. (1982). Estrogen excretion patterns and plasma levels in vegetarian and omnivorous women. *The New England Journal of Medicine*, 307(25), 1542–1547. https://doi.org/10.1056/nejm198212163072502

[87] Gorbach, S. L., & Goldin, B. R. (1987). Diet and the excretion and enterohepatic cycling of estrogens. *Preventive Medicine*, 16(4), 525–531. https://doi.org/10.1016/0091-7435(87)90067-3

[88] Kwa, M., Plottel, C. S., Blaser, M. J., & Adams, S. (2016). The Intestinal Microbiome and Estrogen Receptor-Positive Female Breast Cancer. *Journal of the National Cancer Institute, 108*(8), djw029. https://doi.org/10.1093/jnci/djw029

[89] Sawada, N., Iwasaki, M., Yamaji, T., Shimazu, T., Sasazuki, S., & Tsugane, S. (2015). Fiber intake and risk of subsequent prostate cancer in Japanese men. *The American Journal of Clinical Nutrition*, 101(1), 118–125. https://doi.org/10.3945/ajcn.114.089581

[90] Moosavi, M. A., Haghi, A., Rahmati, M., Taniguchi, H., Mocan, A., Echeverría, J., . . . Atanasov, A. G. (2018). Phytochemicals as potent modulators of autophagy for cancer therapy. *Cancer Letters*, 424, 46–69. https://doi.org/10.1016/j.canlet.2018.02.030

[91] Patra, S., Nayak, R., Patro, S., Pradhan, B., Sahu, B., Behera, C., . . . Jena, M. (2021). Chemical diversity of dietary phytochemicals and their mode of chemoprevention. *Biotechnology Reports*, 30, e00633. https://doi.org/10.1016/j.btre.2021.e00633

[92] Collins, A., Azqueta, A., & Langie, S. a. S. (2012). Effects of micronutrients on DNA repair. *European Journal of Nutrition*, 51(3), 261–279. https://doi.org/10.1007/s00394-012-0318-4

[93] Folkman, J. (2002). Role of angiogenesis in tumor growth and metastasis. *Seminars in Oncology,* 29(6Q), 15–18. https://doi.org/10.1053/sonc.2002.37263

[94] Lišková, A., Koklesová, L., Samec, M., Varghese, E., Abotaleb, M., Samuel, S. M., . . . Kubatka, P. (2020). Implications of flavonoids as potential modulators of cancer neovascularity. *Journal of Cancer Research and Clinical Oncology,* 146(12), 3079–3096. https://doi.org/10.1007/s00432-020-03383-8

[95] Albini, A., Tosetti, F., Li, V. W., Noonan, D. M., & Li, W. W. (2012). Cancer prevention by targeting angiogenesis. *Nature Reviews* Clinical Oncology, 9(9), 498–509. https://doi.org/10.1038/nrclinonc.2012.120

[96] Trumbo, P. R., Schlicker, S. A., Yates, A. A., & Poos, M. I. (2002). Dietary reference intakes for energy, carbohydrate, fiber, fat, fatty acids, cholesterol, protein and amino acids. *Journal of the American Dietetic Association*, 102(11), 1621–1630. https://doi.org/10.1016/s0002-8223(02)90346-9

[97] Goseki, N., Yamazaki, S., Shimojyu, K., Kando, F., Maruyama, M., Endo, M., . . . Takahashi, H. (1995). Synergistic Effect of Methionine-depleting Total Parenteral Nutrition with 5-Fluorouracil on Human Gastric Cancer: A Randomized, Prospective Clinical Trial. *Japanese Journal of Cancer Research*, 86(5), 484–489. https://doi.org/10.1111/j.1349-7006.1995.tb03082.x

[98] Cao, W., Cheng, Q., Fei, X. F., Li, S. F., Yin, H., & Yang, L. (2000). A study of preoperative methionine-depleting parenteral nutrition plus chemotherapy in gastric cancer patients. *World journal of gastroenterology*, 6(2), 255–258. https://doi.org/10.3748/wjg.v6.i2.255

[99] Malumbres, M. (2014). Cyclin-dependent kinases. GenomeBiology.com (London. Print), 15(6), 122. https://doi.org/10.1186/gb4184

[100] Ettl, T., Schulz, D., & Bauer, R. (2022). The renaissance of cyclin dependent kinase inhibitors. *Cancers*, 14(2), 293. https://doi.org/10.3390/cancers14020293

[101] Wallis, K. F., Morehead, L. C., Bird, J., Byrum, S. D., & Miousse, I. R. (2021). Differences in cell death in methionine versus cysteine depletion. *Environmental and Molecular Mutagenesis*, 62(3), 216–226. https://doi.org/10.1002/em.22428

[102] Strekalova, E., Malin, D., Good, D. W., & Cryns, V. L. (2015). Methionine deprivation induces a targetable vulnerability in Triple-Negative breast cancer cells by enhancing TRAIL receptor-2 expression. *Clinical Cancer Research*, 21(12), 2780–2791. https://doi.org/10.1158/1078-0432.ccr-14-2792

[103] Epner, D. E. (2001). Can dietary methionine restriction increase the effectiveness of chemotherapy in treatment of advanced cancer? *Journal of the American College of Nutrition, 20*(sup5), 443S-449S. https://doi.org/10.1080/07315724.2001.10719183

[104] Lu, S., & Epner, D. E. (2000). Molecular mechanisms of cell cycle block by methionine restriction in human prostate cancer cells. *Nutrition and Cancer, 38*(1), 123–130. https://doi.org/10.1207/s15327914nc381_17

[105] Lu, S., Chen, G. L., Ren, C., Kwabi-Addo, B., & Epner, D. E. (2003). Methionine restriction selectively targets thymidylate synthase in prostate cancer cells. *Biochemical Pharmacology, 66*(5), 791–800. https://doi.org/10.1016/s0006-2952(03)00406-4

[106] Kokkinakis, D. M., Liu, X., & Neuner, R. (2005). Modulation of cell cycle and gene expression in pancreatic tumor cell lines by methionine deprivation (methionine stress): implications to the therapy of pancreatic adenocarcinoma. *Molecular Cancer Therapeutics, 4*(9), 1338–1348. https://doi.org/10.1158/1535-7163.mct-05-0141

[107] Locke, E. A., & Latham, G. P. (2002). Building a practically useful theory of goal setting and task motivation: A 35-year odyssey. *American Psychologist, 57*(9), 705–717. https://doi.org/10.1037/0003-066x.57.9.705

CHAPTER 3. UNPOPULAR RESISTANCE: DIABETES

[108] Tokarz, V. L., MacDonald, P. E., & Klip, A. (2018). The cell biology of systemic insulin function. *Journal of Cell Biology, 217*(7), 2273–2289. https://doi.org/10.1083/jcb.201802095

[109] Fletcher, B. J., & Lamendola, C. (2004). Insulin resistance syndrome. *Journal of Cardiovascular Nursing, 19*(5), 339–345. https://doi.org/10.1097/00005082-200409000-00009

[110] Ogawa, W., & Kasuga, M. (2006). [Insulin signaling and pathophysiology of type 2 diabetes mellitus]. *Japanese journal of clinical medicine*, 64(7), 1381–1389. Retrieved from https://pubmed.ncbi.nlm.nih.gov/16838661

[111] Li, T., Ruan, D., Gao, J., Wang, H., & Xu, X. (2018b). [Role of skeletal muscle fat ectopic deposition in insulin resistance induced by high-fat diet]. *Sheng li xue bao : [Acta physiologica Sinica]* , 70(4), 433–444. Retrieved from https://pubmed.ncbi.nlm.nih.gov/30112569

[112] Ritter, O., Jeleník, T., & Roden, M. (2015). Lipid-mediated muscle insulin resistance: different fat, different pathways? *Journal of Molecular Medicine,* 93(8), 831–843. https://doi.org/10.1007/s00109-015-1310-2

[113] Wu, H., & Ballantyne, C. M. (2017). Skeletal muscle inflammation and insulin resistance in obesity. *Journal of Clinical Investigation*, 127(1), 43–54. https://doi.org/10.1172/jci88880

[114] Thomas, D. D., Corkey, B. E., & Istfan, N. W. (2019). Hyperinsulinemia: an early indicator of metabolic dysfunction. *Journal of the Endocrine Society*, 3(9), 1727–1747. https://doi.org/10.1210/js.2019-00065

[115] Arrants, J. E. (1994). Hyperinsulinemia and cardiovascular risk. *Heart & lung : the journal of critical care*, 23(2), 118–4. Retrieved from https://pubmed.ncbi.nlm.nih.gov/8206768

[116] Reaven, G. M. (2003). Insulin Resistance/Compensatory Hyperinsulinemia, essential hypertension, and cardiovascular disease. *The Journal of Clinical Endocrinology & Metabolism*, 88(6), 2399–2403. https://doi.org/10.1210/jc.2003-030087

[117] Stout, R. W. (1996). Hyperinsulinemia and atherosclerosis. *Diabetes,* 45(Supplement_3), S45–S46. https://doi.org/10.2337/diab.45.3.s45

[118] Tasić, I., & Lović, D. (2018). Hypertension and cardiometabolic disease. *Frontiers in Bioscience*, 10(1), 166–174. https://doi.org/10.2741/s506

[119] Da Silva, A. A., Carmo, J. M. D., Li, X., Wang, Z., Mouton, A. J., & Hall, J. E. (2020). Role of hyperinsulinemia and insulin resistance in hypertension: Metabolic Syndrome revisited. *Canadian Journal of Cardiology*, 36(5), 671–682. https://doi.org/10.1016/j.cjca.2020.02.066

[120] Björck, I., & Elmståhl, H. (2003). The glycaemic index: importance of dietary fibre and other food properties. *Proceedings of the Nutrition Society*, 62(1), 201–206. https://doi.org/10.1079/pns2002239

[121] Kaline, K., Bornstein, S. R., Bergmann, A., Hauner, H., & Schwarz, P. E. H. (2007). The Importance and Effect of Dietary Fiber in Diabetes Prevention with Particular Consideration of Whole Grain Products. *Hormone and Metabolic Research*, 39(9), 687–693. https://doi.org/10.1055/s-2007-985811

[122] Salmerón, J. (1997). Dietary fiber, glycemic load, and risk of non—insulin-dependent diabetes mellitus in women. *JAMA*, 277(6), 472. https://doi.org/10.1001/jama.1997.03540300040031

[123] Tan, Q., Li, Y., Li, X., & Zhang, S. (2019). Hyperinsulinemia impairs functions of circulating endothelial progenitor cells. *Acta Diabetologica*, 56(7), 785–795. https://doi.org/10.1007/s00592-019-01314-9

[124] Grandl, G., & Wolfrum, C. (2017). Hemostasis, endothelial stress, inflammation, and the metabolic syndrome. *Seminars in Immunopathology,* 40(2), 215–224. https://doi.org/10.1007/s00281-017-0666-5

[125] Hill, M. A., Yang, Y., Zhang, L., Sun, Z., Jia, G., Parrish, A. R., & Sowers, J. R. (2021). Insulin resistance, cardiovascular stiffening and cardiovascular disease. *Metabolism*, 119, 154766. https://doi.org/10.1016/j.metabol.2021.154766

[126] Julián, M. T., Alonso, N., Ojanguren, I., Pizarro, E., Ballestar, E., & Puig-Domingo, M. (2015). Hepatic glycogenosis: An underdiagnosed complication of diabetes mellitus? *World*

Journal of Diabetes, 6(2), 321. https://doi.org/10.4239/wjd.v6.i2.321

[127] Sears, B., & Perry, M. L. (2015). The role of fatty acids in insulin resistance. *Lipids in Health and Disease*, 14(1). https://doi.org/10.1186/s12944-015-0123-1

[128] Haffner, S. M., Lehto, S., Rönnemaa, T., Pyörälä, K., & Laakso, M. (1998). Mortality from Coronary Heart Disease in Subjects with Type 2 Diabetes and in Nondiabetic Subjects with and without Prior Myocardial Infarction. *The New England Journal of Medicine*, 339(4), 229–234. https://doi.org/10.1056/nejm199807233390404

[129] What is diabetic neuropathy? (2023, February 28). Retrieved from https://www.niddk.nih.gov/health-information/diabetes/overview/preventing-problems/nerve-damage-diabetic-neuropathies/what-is-diabetic-neuropathy

[130] Vinik, A. I., Maser, R. E., Mitchell, B. D., & Freeman, R. (2003). Diabetic autonomic neuropathy. *Diabetes Care*, 26(5), 1553–1579. https://doi.org/10.2337/diacare.26.5.1553

[131] Kazé, A. D., Fonarow, G. C., & Echouffo-Tcheugui, J. B. (2023). Cardiac autonomic dysfunction and risk of silent myocardial infarction among adults with type 2 diabetes. *Journal of the American Heart Association*, 12(20). https://doi.org/10.1161/jaha.123.029814

[132] Djoussé, L., Gaziano, J. M., Buring, J. E., & Lee, I. (2009). Egg consumption and risk of type 2 diabetes in men and women. *Diabetes Care*, 32(2), 295–300. https://doi.org/10.2337/dc08-1271

[133] Wolfram, T., & Ismail-Beigi, F. (2011). Efficacy of High-Fiber diets in the management of Type 2 diabetes mellitus. *Endocrine Practice*, 17(1), 132–142. https://doi.org/10.4158/ep10204.ra

[134] Ojo, O., Feng, Q., Ojo, O. O., & Wang, X. (2020). The Role of Dietary Fibre in Modulating Gut Microbiota Dysbiosis in Patients with Type 2 Diabetes: A Systematic Review and Meta-Analysis of

Randomised Controlled Trials. *Nutrients*, 12(11), 3239. https://doi.org/10.3390/nu12113239

[135] Waddell, I. S., & Orfila, C. (2022). Dietary fiber in the prevention of obesity and obesity-related chronic diseases: From epidemiological evidence to potential molecular mechanisms. *Critical Reviews in Food Science and Nutrition*, 63(27), 8752–8767. https://doi.org/10.1080/10408398.2022.2061909

[136] Pan, J., Zhang, Q., Zhang, C., Yang, W., Liu, H., Lv, Z., . . . Jiao, Z. (2022). Inhibition of dipeptidyl peptidase-4 by flavonoids: Structure–Activity relationship, kinetics and interaction mechanism. *Frontiers in Nutrition*, 9. https://doi.org/10.3389/fnut.2022.892426

[137] De Vadder, F., Kovatcheva-Datchary, P., Goncalves, D., Vinera, J., Zitoun, C., Duchampt, A., . . . Mithieux, G. (2014). Microbiota-Generated metabolites promote metabolic benefits via Gut-Brain neural circuits. *Cell*, 156(1–2), 84–96. https://doi.org/10.1016/j.cell.2013.12.016

[138] Maughan, R., Fallah, J., & Coyle, E. F. (2010). The effects of fasting on metabolism and performance. *British Journal of Sports Medicine*, 44(7), 490–494. https://doi.org/10.1136/bjsm.2010.072181

[139] Musso, G., Gambino, R., & Cassader, M. (2010). Obesity, diabetes, and gut microbiota. *Diabetes Care*, 33(10), 2277–2284. https://doi.org/10.2337/dc10-0556

[140] Hernández, M. a. G., Canfora, E. E., Jocken, J. W. E., & Blaak, E. E. (2019). The Short-Chain fatty acid acetate in body weight control and insulin sensitivity. *Nutrients*, 11(8), 1943. https://doi.org/10.3390/nu11081943

[141] Chávez-Talavera, O., Tailleux, A., Lefèbvre, P., & Staels, B. (2017). Bile acid control of metabolism and inflammation in obesity, Type 2 diabetes, dyslipidemia, and nonalcoholic fatty liver disease. *Gastroenterology*, 152(7), 1679-1694.e3. https://doi.org/10.1053/j.gastro.2017.01.055

[142] Carter, P., Gray, L. J., Troughton, J., Khunti, K., & Davies, M. J. (2010). Fruit and vegetable intake and incidence of type 2 diabetes mellitus: systematic review and meta-analysis. *The BMJ,* 341(aug18 4), c4229. https://doi.org/10.1136/bmj.c4229
[143] Lepretti, M., Martucciello, S., Burgos-Aceves, M. A., Putti, R., & Lionetti, L. (2018). Omega-3 fatty acids and insulin resistance: Focus on the regulation of mitochondria and endoplasmic reticulum stress. *Nutrients,* 10(3), 350. https://doi.org/10.3390/nu10030350
[144] Luévano-Contreras, C., & Chapman-Novakofski, K. (2010). Dietary advanced glycation end products and aging. *Nutrients,* 2(12), 1247–1265. https://doi.org/10.3390/nu2121247
[145] Indyk, D., Bronowicka-Szydełko, A., Gamian, A., & Kuzan, A. (2021). Advanced glycation end products and their receptors in serum of patients with type 2 diabetes. *Scientific Reports,* 11(1). https://doi.org/10.1038/s41598-021-92630-0
[146] Uribarri, J., Woodruff, S., Goodman, S., Cai, W., Chen, X., Pyzik, R., Yong, A., Striker, G. E., & Vlassara, H. (2010). Advanced glycation end products in foods and a practical guide to their reduction in the diet. *Journal of the American Dietetic Association,* 110(6), 911–16.e12. https://doi.org/10.1016/j.jada.2010.03.018
[147] Snelson, M., & Coughlan, M. T. (2019). Dietary Advanced Glycation End Products: Digestion, Metabolism and Modulation of Gut Microbial Ecology. *Nutrients, 11*(2), 215. https://doi.org/10.3390/nu11020215
[148] Uribarri, J., Del Castillo, M. D., De La Maza, M. P., Filip, R., Gugliucci, A., Luévano-Contreras, C., . . . Garay-Sevilla, M. E. (2015). Dietary Advanced glycation end products and their role in health and disease. *Advances in Nutrition,* 6(4), 461–473. https://doi.org/10.3945/an.115.008433
[149] Bahour, N., Cortez, B., Hui, P., Shah, H., Doria, A., & Aguayo-Mazzucato, C. (2021). Diabetes mellitus correlates with

increased biological age as indicated by clinical biomarkers. *GeroScience*, 44(1), 415–427. https://doi.org/10.1007/s11357-021-00469-0

[150] Yaffe, K., Kanaya, A. M., Lindquist, K., Simonsick, E. M., Harris, T. B., Shorr, R. I., . . . Newman, A. B. (2004). The metabolic syndrome, inflammation, and risk of cognitive decline. *JAMA*, *292*(18), 2237. https://doi.org/10.1001/jama.292.18.2237

[151] Kim, B., & Feldman, E. L. (2015). Insulin resistance as a key link for the increased risk of cognitive impairment in the metabolic syndrome. *Experimental & Molecular Medicine*, 47(3), e149. https://doi.org/10.1038/emm.2015.3

[152] Nelson, P. T., Smith, C. D., Abner, E. L., Schmitt, F. A., Scheff, S. W., Davis, G. J., . . . Markesbery, W. R. (2009). Human cerebral neuropathology of Type 2 diabetes mellitus. Biochimica Et Biophysica Acta (BBA) - *Molecular Basis of Disease*, 1792(5), 454–469. https://doi.org/10.1016/j.bbadis.2008.08.005

[153] Etchegoyen, M., Nobile, M. H., Báez, F., Posesorski, B., González, J., Lago, N., . . . Otero-Losada, M. (2018). *Metabolic syndrome and neuroprotection*. Frontiers in Neuroscience, 12. https://doi.org/10.3389/fnins.2018.00196

[154] Yau, P. L., Castro, B. M. G., Tagani, A., Tsui, W., & Convit, A. (2012). Obesity and metabolic syndrome and functional and structural brain impairments in adolescence. *Pediatrics,* 130(4), e856–e864. https://doi.org/10.1542/peds.2012-0324

[155] Michailidis, M., Moraitou, D., Tata, D. A., Kalinderi, K., Papamitsou, T., & Papaliagkas, V. (2022). Alzheimer's Disease as Type 3 Diabetes: Common Pathophysiological Mechanisms between Alzheimer's Disease and Type 2 Diabetes. *International Journal of Molecular Sciences*, 23(5), 2687. https://doi.org/10.3390/ijms23052687

[156] Nguyen, T. T., Ta, Q. T. H., Nguyen, T. K. O., Nguyen, T. T. D., & Van Giau, V. (2020). Type 3 diabetes and its role implications in

Alzheimer's disease. *International Journal of Molecular Sciences*, 21(9), 3165. https://doi.org/10.3390/ijms21093165

[157] Janoutová, J., Machaczka, O., Zatloukalová, A., & Janout, V. (2022). Is Alzheimer's disease a type 3 diabetes? A review. *Central European Journal of Public Health*, 30(3), 139–143. https://doi.org/10.21101/cejph.a7238

[158] Arnold, S. E., Arvanitakis, Z., Macauley, S. L., Koenig, A. M., Wang, H. Y., Ahima, R. S., . . . Nathan, D. M. (2018). Brain insulin resistance in type 2 diabetes and Alzheimer disease: concepts and conundrums. *Nature Reviews Neurology*, 14(3), 168–181. https://doi.org/10.1038/nrneurol.2017.185

[159] Ahmed, S., Mahmood, Z., & Zahid, S. (2015). Linking insulin with Alzheimer's disease: emergence as type III diabetes. *Neurological Sciences*, 36(10), 1763–1769. https://doi.org/10.1007/s10072-015-2352-5

[160] Mergenthaler, P., Lindauer, U., Dienel, G. A., & Meisel, A. (2013). Sugar for the brain: the role of glucose in physiological and pathological brain function. *Trends in Neurosciences*, 36(10), 587–597. https://doi.org/10.1016/j.tins.2013.07.001

[161] Kirchhoff, B. A., Lugar, H. M., Smith, S. E., Meyer, E. G., Perantie, D. C., Kolody, B. C., . . . Hershey, T. (2013). Hypoglycaemia-induced changes in regional brain volume and memory function. *Diabetic Medicine*, 30(4). https://doi.org/10.1111/dme.12135

[162] De Natale, C., Annuzzi, G., Bozzetto, L., Mazzarella, R., Costabile, G., Ciano, O., . . . Rivellese, A. A. (2009). Effects of a Plant-Based High-Carbohydrate/High-Fiber diet versus High–Monounsaturated Fat/Low-Carbohydrate diet on postprandial lipids in Type 2 diabetic patients. *Diabetes Care*, 32(12), 2168–2173. https://doi.org/10.2337/dc09-0266

[163] Aune, D., Ursin, G., & Veierød, M. B. (2009). Meat consumption and the risk of type 2 diabetes: a systematic review

and meta-analysis of cohort studies. *Diabetologia,* 52(11), 2277–2287. https://doi.org/10.1007/s00125-009-1481-x
[164] Barnard, N. D., Cohen, J., Jenkins, D., Turner-McGrievy, G., Gloede, L., Green, A., & Ferdowsian, H. (2009). A low-fat vegan diet and a conventional diabetes diet in the treatment of type 2 diabetes: a randomized, controlled, 74-wk clinical trial. *The American Journal of Clinical Nutrition,* 89(5), 1588S-1596S. https://doi.org/10.3945/ajcn.2009.26736h
[165] Fung, T. T., Schulze, M. B., Manson, J. E., Willett, W. C., & Hu, F. B. (2004). Dietary patterns, meat intake, and the risk of type 2 diabetes in women. *Archives of Internal Medicine,* 164(20), 2235. https://doi.org/10.1001/archinte.164.20.2235
[166] Kahleová, H., Matoulek, M., Malínská, H., Oliyarnik, O., Kazdová, L., Neškudla, T., . . . Pelikánová, T. (2011). Vegetarian diet improves insulin resistance and oxidative stress markers more than conventional diet in subjects with Type 2 diabetes. *Diabetic Medicine,* 28(5), 549–559. https://doi.org/10.1111/j.1464-5491.2010.03209.x
[167] Tonstad, S., Butler, T., Yan, R., & Fraser, G. E. (2009). Type of vegetarian diet, body weight, and prevalence of type 2 diabetes. *Diabetes Care,* 32(5), 791–796. https://doi.org/10.2337/dc08-1886
[168] Vang, A., Singh, P. N., Lee, J., Haddad, E., & Brinegar, C. H. (2008). Meats, Processed Meats, Obesity, Weight Gain and Occurrence of Diabetes among Adults: Findings from Adventist Health Studies. *Annals of Nutrition and Metabolism,* 52(2), 96–104. https://doi.org/10.1159/000121365
[169] Thomas, T. T., & Pfeiffer, A. F. H. (2012). Foods for the prevention of diabetes: how do they work? *Diabetes/Metabolism Research and Reviews,* 28(1), 25–49. https://doi.org/10.1002/dmrr.1229
[170] McMacken, M., & Shah, S. R. (2017). A plant-based diet for the prevention and treatment of type 2 diabetes. *Journal of*

geriatric cardiology : JGC, 14(5), 342–354.
https://doi.org/10.11909/j.issn.1671-5411.2017.05.009
[171] Jardine, M., Kahleová, H., Levin, S., Ali, Z., Trapp, C., & Barnard, N. D. (2021). Perspective: Plant-Based Eating Pattern for Type 2 Diabetes Prevention and Treatment: Efficacy, mechanisms, and practical considerations. *Advances in Nutrition*, 12(6), 2045–2055. https://doi.org/10.1093/advances/nmab063
[172] Mokdad, A. H., Ballestros, K., Echko, M., Glenn, S., Olsen, H. E., Mullany, E. C., . . . Murray, C. J. L. (2018). The State of US Health, 1990-2016. *JAMA*, 319(14), 1444.
https://doi.org/10.1001/jama.2018.0158

CHAPTER 4. UNTANGLING THE GORDIAN KNOT: HEART HEALTH

[173] Badimon, L., & Vilahur, G. (2014). Thrombosis formation on atherosclerotic lesions and plaque rupture. *Journal of Internal Medicine*, 276(6), 618–632. https://doi.org/10.1111/joim.12296
[174] Taleb, S. (2016). Inflammation in atherosclerosis. *Archives of Cardiovascular Diseases*, 109(12), 708–715.
https://doi.org/10.1016/j.acvd.2016.04.002
[175] Alberts, B. (2002). Blood vessels and endothelial cells. Retrieved from https://www.ncbi.nlm.nih.gov/books/NBK26848/
[176] Fung, T. T., McCullough, M. L., Newby, P. K., Manson, J. E., Meigs, J. B., Rifai, N., . . . Hu, F. B. (2005). Diet-quality scores and plasma concentrations of markers of inflammation and endothelial dysfunction. *The American Journal of Clinical Nutrition*, 82(1), 163–173. https://doi.org/10.1093/ajcn.82.1.163
[177] Patel, H., Chandra, S., Alexander, S., Soble, J. S., & Williams, K. A. (2017). Plant-Based nutrition: an essential component of cardiovascular disease prevention and management. *Current Cardiology Reports*, 19(10). https://doi.org/10.1007/s11886-017-0909-z

[178] Kim, H., Caulfield, L. E., García-Larsen, V., Steffen, L. M., Coresh, J., & Rebholz, C. M. (2019). Plant-Based diets are associated with a lower risk of incident cardiovascular disease, cardiovascular disease mortality, and All-Cause mortality in a general population of Middle-Aged adults. *Journal of the American Heart Association,* 8(16). https://doi.org/10.1161/jaha.119.012865

[179] Gan, Z. H., Cheong, H. C., Tu, Y., & Kuo, P. (2021). Association between Plant-Based Dietary Patterns and Risk of Cardiovascular Disease: A Systematic Review and Meta-Analysis of Prospective Cohort Studies. *Nutrients,* 13(11), 3952. https://doi.org/10.3390/nu13113952

[180] Mishra, S., Xu, J., Agarwal, U., Gonzales, J., Levin, S., & Barnard, N. D. (2013). A multicenter randomized controlled trial of a plant-based nutrition program to reduce body weight and cardiovascular risk in the corporate setting: the GEICO study. *European Journal of Clinical Nutrition,* 67(7), 718–724. https://doi.org/10.1038/ejcn.2013.92

[181] Kahleová, H., Levin, S., & Barnard, N. D. (2018). Vegetarian dietary patterns and cardiovascular disease. *Progress in Cardiovascular Diseases,* 61(1), 54–61. https://doi.org/10.1016/j.pcad.2018.05.002

[182] Salehin, S., Rasmussen, P. R., Mai, S., Mushtaq, M., Agarwal, M., Hasan, S. M., . . . Khalife, W. (2023). Plant based diet and its effect on cardiovascular disease. *International Journal of Environmental Research and Public Health,* 20(4), 3337. https://doi.org/10.3390/ijerph20043337

[183] Delgado-Velandía, M., Maroto-Rodríguez, J., Ortolá, R., García-Esquinas, E., Rodríguez-Artalejo, F., & Sotos-Prieto, M. (2022). Plant-Based diets and all-cause and cardiovascular mortality in a nationwide cohort in Spain. *Mayo Clinic Proceedings,* 97(11), 2005–2015. https://doi.org/10.1016/j.mayocp.2022.06.008

[184] Hemler, E. C., & Hu, F. B. (2019). Plant-Based diets for personal, population, and planetary health. *Advances in Nutrition*, 10, S275–S283. https://doi.org/10.1093/advances/nmy117

[185] Peña-Jorquera, H., Cid-Jofré, V., Landaeta-Díaz, L., Petermann-Rocha, F., Martorell, M., Zbinden-Foncea, H., . . . Cristi-Montero, C. (2023). Plant-Based Nutrition: Exploring Health benefits for Atherosclerosis, Chronic Diseases, and Metabolic Syndrome—A Comprehensive review. *Nutrients*, 15(14), 3244. https://doi.org/10.3390/nu15143244

[186] Dehghan, M., Mente, A., Teo, K., Gao, P., Sleight, P., Dagenais, G. R., . . . Yusuf, S. (2012). Relationship between healthy diet and risk of cardiovascular disease among patients on drug therapies for secondary prevention. *Circulation*, 126(23), 2705–2712. https://doi.org/10.1161/circulationaha.112.103234

[187] Hennig, B., Diana, J. N., Toborek, M., & McClain, C. J. (1994). Influence of nutrients and cytokines on endothelial cell metabolism. *Journal of the American College of Nutrition*, 13(3), 224–231. https://doi.org/10.1080/07315724.1994.10718401

[188] Hennig, B., Toborek, M., & McClain, C. J. (2001). High-Energy diets, fatty acids and endothelial cell function: Implications for atherosclerosis. *Journal of the American College of Nutrition*, 20(2), 97–105. https://doi.org/10.1080/07315724.2001.10719021

[189] Mao, C., Li, D., Zhou, E., Zhang, J., Wang, C., & Xue, C. (2021). Nicotine exacerbates atherosclerosis through a macrophage-mediated endothelial injury pathway. *Aging*, 13(5), 7627–7643. https://doi.org/10.18632/aging.202660

[190] Corona, G., Rastrelli, G., Isidori, A. M., Pivonello, R., Bettocchi, C., Reisman, Y., . . . Maggi, M. (2020). Erectile dysfunction and cardiovascular risk: a review of current findings. *Expert Review of Cardiovascular Therapy*, 18(3), 155–164. https://doi.org/10.1080/14779072.2020.1745632

[191] Nehra, A., Jackson, G., Miner, M., Billups, K. L., Burnett, A. L., Buvat, J., . . . Wu, F. C. W. (2013). Diagnosis and treatment of erectile dysfunction for reduction of cardiovascular risk. *The Journal of Urology,* 189(6), 2031–2038. https://doi.org/10.1016/j.juro.2012.12.107

[192] Stary, H. C., Chandler, A. B., Glagov, S., Guyton, J. R., Insull, W., Rosenfeld, M. E., . . . Wissler, R. W. (1994). A definition of initial, fatty streak, and intermediate lesions of atherosclerosis. A report from the Committee on Vascular Lesions of the Council on Arteriosclerosis, American Heart Association. *Circulation,* 89(5), 2462–2478. https://doi.org/10.1161/01.cir.89.5.2462

[193] Rosenfeld, M. E. (2000). An overview of the evolution of the atherosclerotic plaque: from fatty streak to plaque rupture and thrombosis. *Zeitschrift Fur Kardiologie,* 89(S7), VII2–VII6. https://doi.org/10.1007/s003920070045

[194] Stocco, D. M. (2000). Intramitochondrial cholesterol transfer. Biochimica Et Biophysica Acta (BBA) - *Molecular and Cell Biology of Lipids,* 1486(1), 184–197. https://doi.org/10.1016/s1388-1981(00)00056-1

[195] Cerqueira, N. M. F. S. A., Oliveira, E. F., Gesto, D., Santos-Martins, D., Moreira, C., Moorthy, H. N., . . . Fernandes, P. A. (2016). Cholesterol Biosynthesis: A Mechanistic Overview. *Biochemistry,* 55(39), 5483–5506. https://doi.org/10.1021/acs.biochem.6b00342

[196] Wang, N., & Westerterp, M. (2020). ABC transporters, cholesterol efflux, and implications for cardiovascular diseases. *Advances in Experimental Medicine and Biology* (pp. 67–83). https://doi.org/10.1007/978-981-15-6082-8_6

[197] Li, G., Gu, H., & Zhang, D. (2013). ATP-binding cassette transporters and cholesterol translocation. *IUBMB Life,* 65(6), 505–512. https://doi.org/10.1002/iub.1165

[198] Schmitz, G., & Kaminski, W. E. (2001). ABC transporters and cholesterol metabolism. *Frontiers in Bioscience*, 6(1), d505. https://doi.org/10.2741/schmitz

[199] Plösch, T., Kosters, A., Groen, A. K., & Kuipers, F. (2005). The ABC of Hepatic and intestinal cholesterol transport. *Handbook of experimental pharmacology* (pp. 465–482). https://doi.org/10.1007/3-540-27661-0_17

[200] Reeskamp, L. F., Meessen, E. C. E., & Groen, A. K. (2018). Transintestinal cholesterol excretion in humans. *Current Opinion in Lipidology*, 29(1), 10–17. https://doi.org/10.1097/mol.0000000000000473

[201] Ioannou, G. N. (2016). The role of cholesterol in the pathogenesis of NASH. *Trends in Endocrinology and Metabolism*, 27(2), 84–95. https://doi.org/10.1016/j.tem.2015.11.008

[202] Chen, Y., Chen, Y., Zhao, L., Mei, M., Li, Q., Huang, A., . . . Ruan, X. Z. (2012). Inflammatory stress exacerbates hepatic cholesterol accumulation via disrupting cellular cholesterol export. *Journal of Gastroenterology and Hepatology*, 27(5), 974–984. https://doi.org/10.1111/j.1440-1746.2011.06986.x

[203] Curley, S., Gall, J., Byrne, R., Yvan-Charvet, L., & McGillicuddy, F. C. (2020). Metabolic Inflammation in Obesity—At the Crossroads between Fatty Acid and Cholesterol Metabolism. *Molecular Nutrition & Food Research*, 65(1). https://doi.org/10.1002/mnfr.201900482

[204] Tsoupras, A., & Lordan, R. (2018). Inflammation, not Cholesterol, Is a Cause of Chronic Disease. *Nutrients*, 10(5), 604. https://doi.org/10.3390/nu10050604

[205] Simopoulos, A. P. (2016). An increase in the Omega-6/Omega-3 fatty acid ratio increases the risk for obesity. *Nutrients*, 8(3), 128. https://doi.org/10.3390/nu8030128

[206] Parikh, M., Maddaford, T. G., Austria, J. A., Aliani, M., Netticadan, T., & Pierce, G. N. (2019). Dietary flaxseed as a

strategy for improving human health. *Nutrients*, 11(5), 1171. https://doi.org/10.3390/nu11051171

[207] Giugliano, D., Ceriello, A., & Esposito, K. (2006). The effects of diet on inflammation. *Journal of the American College of Cardiology*, 48(4), 677–685. https://doi.org/10.1016/j.jacc.2006.03.052

[208] Aune, D. (2019). Plant foods, antioxidant biomarkers, and the risk of cardiovascular disease, cancer, and mortality: A review of the evidence. *Advances in Nutrition*, 10, S404–S421. https://doi.org/10.1093/advances/nmz042

[209] Tribble, D. L. (1999). Antioxidant consumption and risk of coronary heart disease: Emphasis on vitamin C, vitamin E, and B-Carotene. *Circulation*, 99(4), 591–595. https://doi.org/10.1161/01.cir.99.4.591

[210] Strong, J. P., Malcom, G. T., Newman, W. P., & Oalmann, M. C. (1992). Early lesions of atherosclerosis in Childhood and Youth: natural history and risk factors. *Journal of the American College of Nutrition,* 11(sup1), 51S-54S. https://doi.org/10.1080/07315724.1992.10737984

[211] Gątarek, P., & Kałużna–Czaplińska, J. (2021). Trimethylamine N-oxide (TMAO) in human health. *Excli Journal*, 20, 301–319. https://doi.org/10.17179/excli2020-3239

[212] Vourakis, M., Mayer, G., & Rousseau, G. (2021). The role of gut microbiota on cholesterol metabolism in atherosclerosis. *International Journal of Molecular Sciences*, 22(15), 8074. https://doi.org/10.3390/ijms22158074

[213] Koeth, R. A., Wang, Z., Levison, B. S., Buffa, J. A., Org, E., Sheehy, B., . . . Hazen, S. L. (2013). Intestinal microbiota metabolism of l-carnitine, a nutrient in red meat, promotes atherosclerosis. *Nature Medicine*, 19(5), 576–585. https://doi.org/10.1038/nm.3145

[214] Maurice, J., & Manousou, P. (2018). Non-alcoholic fatty liver disease. *Clinical Medicine*, 18(3), 245–250. https://doi.org/10.7861/clinmedicine.18-3-245

[215] Skippon, W. (2013). The animal health and welfare consequences of foie gras production. PubMed. Retrieved from https://pubmed.ncbi.nlm.nih.gov/24082171

[216] American Veterinary Medical Association. (2014, May). Literature Review on the Welfare Implications of Foie Gras Production. Retrieved from https://www.avma.org/sites/default/files/resources/foie_gras_bgnd.pdf

[217] Cortés, B., Núñez, I., Cofán, M., Gilabert, R., Pérez-Heras, A., Casals, E., Deulofeu, R., & Ros, E. (2006). Acute effects of high-fat meals enriched with walnuts or olive oil on postprandial endothelial function. *Journal of the American College of Cardiology*, 48(8), 1666–1671. https://doi.org/10.1016/j.jacc.2006.06.057

[218] Ornish, D., Brown, S. C., Billings, J. H., Scherwitz, L., Armstrong, W., Ports, T. A., . . . Brand, R. (1990). Can lifestyle changes reverse coronary heart disease? *The Lancet*, 336(8708), 129–133. https://doi.org/10.1016/0140-6736(90)91656-u

[219] Esselstyn, C. B. (2001). Resolving the coronary artery disease epidemic through Plant-Based Nutrition. *Preventive Cardiology*, 4(4), 171–177. https://doi.org/10.1111/j.1520037x.2001.00538.x

[220] Esselstyn, C. B. (1999). Updating a 12-year experience with arrest and reversal therapy for coronary heart disease (an overdue requiem for palliative cardiology). *The American Journal of Cardiology*, 84(3), 339–341. https://doi.org/10.1016/s0002-9149(99)00290-8

[221] Ornish, D., Scherwitz, L., Billings, J. H., Gould, K. L., Merritt, T. A., Sparler, S., . . . Brand, R. (1998). Intensive lifestyle changes for reversal of coronary heart disease. *JAMA*, 280(23), 2001. https://doi.org/10.1001/jama.280.23.2001

[222] Haskell, W. L., Alderman, E. L., Fair, J. M., Maron, D. J., Mackey, S., Superko, H. R., . . . Krauss, R. M. (1994). Effects of intensive multiple risk factor reduction on coronary atherosclerosis and clinical cardiac events in men and women with coronary artery disease. The Stanford Coronary Risk Intervention Project (SCRIP). *Circulation*, 89(3), 975–990. https://doi.org/10.1161/01.cir.89.3.975

[223] Ma, X., Chen, Q., Pu, Y., Guo, M., Jiang, Z., Huang, W., . . . Xu, Y. (2020). Skipping breakfast is associated with overweight and obesity: A systematic review and meta-analysis. *Obesity Research & Clinical Practice,* 14(1), 1–8. https://doi.org/10.1016/j.orcp.2019.12.002

[224] Dulloo, A. G. (2021). Physiology of weight regain: Lessons from the classic Minnesota Starvation Experiment on human body composition regulation. *Obesity Reviews*, 22(S2). https://doi.org/10.1111/obr.13189

[225] Kojima, M., & Kangawa, K. (2005). Ghrelin: Structure and function. *Physiological Reviews*, 85(2), 495–522. https://doi.org/10.1152/physrev.00012.2004

[226] Cahill, L. E., Chiuve, S. E., Mekary, R. A., Jensen, M. K., Flint, A., Hu, F. B., & Rimm, E. B. (2013). Prospective study of breakfast eating and incident coronary heart disease in a cohort of male US health professionals. *Circulation,* 128(4), 337–343. https://doi.org/10.1161/circulationaha.113.001474

[227] Malik, V., Li, Y., Tobias, D. K., Pan, A., & Hu, F. B. (2016). Dietary protein intake and risk of type 2 diabetes in US men and women. *American Journal of Epidemiology*, 183(8), 715–728. https://doi.org/10.1093/aje/kwv268

[228] Whelan, W. J., Ghanchi, H., & Ricciardi, M. J. (2010). Protein causes a glycemic response. *IUBMB Life*, 62(6), 477–479. https://doi.org/10.1002/iub.333

[229] Perkins, J. M., Joy, N. G., Tate, D. B., & Davis, S. N. (2015). Acute effects of hyperinsulinemia and hyperglycemia on vascular

inflammatory biomarkers and endothelial function in overweight and obese humans. *American Journal of Physiology-endocrinology and Metabolism*, 309(2), E168–E176. https://doi.org/10.1152/ajpendo.00064.2015

[230] Sun, Y., Liu, B., Snetselaar, L., Wallace, R. B., Shadyab, A. H., Kroenke, C. H., . . . Bao, W. (2021). Association of major dietary protein Sources with All-Cause and Cause-Specific Mortality: Prospective Cohort study. *Journal of the American Heart Association,* 10(5). https://doi.org/10.1161/jaha.119.015553

[231] Forde, C. G., & De Graaf, K. (2022). Influence of sensory properties in moderating eating behaviors and food intake. *Frontiers in Nutrition,* 9. https://doi.org/10.3389/fnut.2022.841444

[232] Food Data Central. (n.d.). Retrieved from https://fdc.nal.usda.gov/fdc-app.html#/food-details/171279/nutrients

[233] Calorie calculator. (2022, November 29). Retrieved from https://www.mayoclinic.org/healthy-lifestyle/weight-loss/in-depth/calorie-calculator/itt-20402304

[234] Millward, D. J. (1999). Meat or wheat for the next millennium? *Proceedings of the Nutrition Society,* 58(2), 209–210. https://doi.org/10.1017/s0029665199000294

[235] Parker, H., & Vadiveloo, M. (2019). Diet quality of vegetarian diets compared with nonvegetarian diets: a systematic review. *Nutrition Reviews*, 77(3), 144–160. https://doi.org/10.1093/nutrit/nuy067

[236] Craig, W. J., & Mangels, A. R. (2009). Position of the American Dietetic Association: Vegetarian diets. *Journal of the American Dietetic Association,* 109(7), 1266–1282. https://doi.org/10.1016/j.jada.2009.05.027

[237] Lynch, H., Wharton, C., & Johnston, C. S. (2016). Cardiorespiratory Fitness and Peak Torque Differences between

Vegetarian and Omnivore Endurance Athletes: A Cross-Sectional Study. *Nutrients*, 8(11), 726. https://doi.org/10.3390/nu8110726
[238] Boutros, G., Landry-Duval, M., Garzón, M., & Karelis, A. D. (2020). Is a vegan diet detrimental to endurance and muscle strength? *European Journal of Clinical Nutrition*, 74(11), 1550–1555. https://doi.org/10.1038/s41430-020-0639-y
[239] Podlogar, T., & Wallis, G. A. (2022). New horizons in carbohydrate research and application for endurance athletes. *Sports Medicine*, 52(S1), 5–23. https://doi.org/10.1007/s40279-022-01757-1

CHAPTER 5. AGING: WHY THE RUSH TO AGE?

[240] Li, L., Zhuang, Y., Zou, X., Chen, M., Cui, B., Ye, J., & Cheng, Y. (2023). Advanced Glycation End Products: A comprehensive review of their detection and occurrence in food. *Foods*, 12(11), 2103. https://doi.org/10.3390/foods12112103
[241] Willcox, D. C., Willcox, B. J., Todoriki, H., & Suzuki, M. (2009). The Okinawan Diet: health implications of a Low-Calorie, Nutrient-Dense, Antioxidant-Rich dietary pattern low in glycemic load. *Journal of the American College of Nutrition*, 28(sup4), 500S-516S. https://doi.org/10.1080/07315724.2009.10718117
[242] Lev-Ran, A. (2001). Human obesity: an evolutionary approach to understanding our bulging waistline. *Diabetes/Metabolism Research and Reviews*, 17(5), 347–362. https://doi.org/10.1002/dmrr.230
[243] Danby, F. W. (2010). Nutrition and aging skin: sugar and glycation. *Clinics in Dermatology*, 28(4), 409–411. https://doi.org/10.1016/j.clindermatol.2010.03.018
[244] Katta, R., Sánchez, A., & Tantry, E. (2020b). An Anti-Wrinkle Diet: Nutritional Strategies to Combat Oxidation, Inflammation and Glycation. *Skin Therapy Letter*, 25(2), 3–7.

[245] Vatner, S. F., Zhang, J., Oydanich, M., Berkman, T., Naftalovich, R., & Vatner, D. E. (2020). Healthful aging mediated by inhibition of oxidative stress. *Ageing Research Reviews*, 64, 101194. https://doi.org/10.1016/j.arr.2020.101194
[246] Finkel, T., & Holbrook, N. J. (2000). Oxidants, oxidative stress and the biology of ageing. *Nature*, 408(6809), 239–247. https://doi.org/10.1038/35041687
[247] Turnbull, O., Homer, M., & Ensaff, H. (2021). Food insecurity: Its prevalence and relationship to fruit and vegetable consumption. *Journal of Human Nutrition and Dietetics*, 34(5), 849–857. https://doi.org/10.1111/jhn.12866
[248] Gerritsen, R. J. S., & Band, G. P. H. (2018). Breath of Life: the respiratory vagal stimulation model of contemplative activity. *Frontiers in Human Neuroscience*, 12. https://doi.org/10.3389/fnhum.2018.00397
[249] Louie, D., Brook, K., & Frates, E. P. (2016). The laughter prescription. *American Journal of Lifestyle Medicine*, 10(4), 262–267. https://doi.org/10.1177/1559827614550279
[250] Wakefield, J. R. H., Këllezi, B., Stevenson, C., McNamara, N., Bowe, M., Wilson, I. S., . . . Mair, E. (2020). Social Prescribing as 'Social Cure': A longitudinal study of the health benefits of social connectedness within a Social Prescribing pathway. *Journal of Health Psychology*, 27(2), 386–396. https://doi.org/10.1177/1359105320944991
[251] O'Rourke, H. M., & Sidani, S. (2017). Definition, Determinants, and Outcomes of Social Connectedness for Older Adults: A scoping review. *Journal of Gerontological Nursing*, 43(7), 43–52. https://doi.org/10.3928/00989134-20170223-03
[252] Lamblin, M., Murawski, C., Whittle, S., & Fornito, A. (2017). Social connectedness, mental health and the adolescent brain. *Neuroscience & Biobehavioral Reviews*, 80, 57–68. https://doi.org/10.1016/j.neubiorev.2017.05.010

[253] Berkman, L. F., & Syme, S. L. (1979). Social networks, host resistance, and mortality: a nine-year follow-up study of Alameda County residents. *American journal of epidemiology*, 109(2), 186–204. https://doi.org/10.1093/oxfordjournals.aje.a112674

[254] House, J. S., Landis, K. R., & Umberson, D. (1988). Social relationships and health. *Science*, 241(4865), 540–545. https://doi.org/10.1126/science.3399889

[255] Ruberman, W., Weinblatt, E., Goldberg, J. D., & Chaudhary, B. S. (1984). Psychosocial Influences on Mortality after Myocardial Infarction. *The New England Journal of Medicine*, 311(9), 552–559. https://doi.org/10.1056/nejm198408303110902

[256] Yang, Y. C., Schorpp, K. M., & Harris, K. M. (2014). Social support, social strain and inflammation: Evidence from a national longitudinal study of U.S. adults. *Social Science & Medicine*, 107, 124–135. https://doi.org/10.1016/j.socscimed.2014.02.013

[257] Rico-Uribe, L. A., Caballero, F. F., Martín-María, N., Cabello, M., Ayuso-Mateos, J. L., & Miret, M. (2018). Association of loneliness with all-cause mortality: A meta-analysis. *PLOS ONE*, 13(1), e0190033. https://doi.org/10.1371/journal.pone.0190033

[258] Morgan K N, Tromborg C T. (2007). Sources of stress in captivity, *Applied Animal Behaviour Science*. 102 (3–4) 262-302. https://doi.org/10.1016/j.applanim.2006.05.032

[259] Oswald, V., Vanhaudenhuyse, A., Annen, J., Martial, C., Bicego, A. Y., Rousseaux, F., ... Gosseries, O. (2023). Autonomic nervous system modulation during self-induced non-ordinary states of consciousness. *Scientific Reports*, 13(1). https://doi.org/10.1038/s41598-023-42393-7

CHAPTER 6. THE SIXTH SENSE ORGAN: GUT FEELING

[260] Khan, R., Kuenzig, M. E., & Benchimol, E. I. (2023). Epidemiology of Pediatric Inflammatory Bowel Disease.

Gastroenterology Clinics of North America, 52(3), 483–496. https://doi.org/10.1016/j.gtc.2023.05.001

[261] Ng, S. C., Shi, H., Hamidi, N., Underwood, F. E., Tang, W., Benchimol, E. I., . . . Kaplan, G. G. (2017). Worldwide incidence and prevalence of inflammatory bowel disease in the 21st century: a systematic review of population-based studies. *The Lancet*, 390(10114), 2769–2778. https://doi.org/10.1016/s0140-6736(17)32448-0

[262] De Medina, F. S., Romero-Calvo, I., Mascaraque, C., & Martínez-Augustin, O. (2014). Intestinal inflammation and mucosal barrier function. *Inflammatory Bowel Diseases*, 20(12), 2394–2404. https://doi.org/10.1097/mib.0000000000000204

[263] Zhang, Y., & Li, Y. (2014). Inflammatory bowel disease: Pathogenesis. *World Journal of Gastroenterology*, 20(1), 91. https://doi.org/10.3748/wjg.v20.i1.91

[264] Peixoto, P., Cartron, P., Sérandour, A. A., & Hervouet, É. (2020). From 1957 to Nowadays: A Brief History of Epigenetics. *International Journal of Molecular Sciences*, 21(20), 7571. https://doi.org/10.3390/ijms21207571

[265] Orholm, M., Binder, V., Sørensen, T. I. A., Rasmussen, L. P., & Kyvik, K. O. (2000). Concordance of Inflammatory Bowel Disease among Danish Twins: Results of a Nationwide Study. *Scandinavian Journal of Gastroenterology,* 35(10), 1075–1081. https://doi.org/10.1080/003655200451207

[266] Borowitz, S. M. (2023). The epidemiology of inflammatory bowel disease: Clues to pathogenesis? *Frontiers in Pediatrics*, 10. https://doi.org/10.3389/fped.2022.1103713

[267] Agrawal, M., & Jess, T. (2022). Implications of the changing epidemiology of inflammatory bowel disease in a changing world. *United European Gastroenterology Journal*, 10(10), 1113–1120. https://doi.org/10.1002/ueg2.12317

[268] Kaplan, G. G., & Ng, S. C. (2017). Understanding and preventing the global increase of inflammatory bowel disease.

Gastroenterology, 152(2), 313-321.e2. https://doi.org/10.1053/j.gastro.2016.10.020

[269] Ahmed, S., Newton, P., Ojo, O., & Dibley, L. (2021). Experiences of ethnic minority patients who are living with a primary chronic bowel condition: a systematic scoping review with narrative synthesis. *BMC Gastroenterology,* 21(1). https://doi.org/10.1186/s12876-021-01857-8

[270] Agrawal, M., Burisch, J., Colombel, J., & Shah, S. C. (2019). Viewpoint: Inflammatory Bowel Diseases among Immigrants From Low- to High-Incidence Countries: Opportunities and Considerations. *Journal of Crohn's and Colitis*, 14(2), 267–273. https://doi.org/10.1093/ecco-jcc/jjz139

[271] Hills, R. D., Pontefract, B., Mishcon, H. R., Black, C. A., Sutton, S. C., & Theberge, C. R. (2019). Gut microbiome: Profound implications for diet and disease. *Nutrients*, 11(7), 1613. https://doi.org/10.3390/nu11071613

[272] Wong, J. M. W., De Souza, R. J., Kendall, C. W., Emam, A., & Jenkins, D. (2006). Colonic health: fermentation and short chain fatty acids. *Journal of Clinical Gastroenterology*, 40(3), 235–243. https://doi.org/10.1097/00004836-200603000-00015

[273] Trakman, G. L., Fehily, S., Basnayake, C., Hamilton, A. L., Russell, E., Wilson-O'Brien, A., & Kamm, M. A. (2021). Diet and gut microbiome in gastrointestinal disease. *Journal of Gastroenterology and Hepatology,* 37(2), 237–245. https://doi.org/10.1111/jgh.15728

[274] David, L. A., Maurice, C. F., Carmody, R. N., Gootenberg, D. B., Button, J. E., Wolfe, B. E., . . . Turnbaugh, P. J. (2013). Diet rapidly and reproducibly alters the human gut microbiome. *Nature,* 505(7484), 559–563. https://doi.org/10.1038/nature12820

[275] Gracie, D. J., Hamlin, P. J., & Ford, A. C. (2019). The influence of the brain–gut axis in inflammatory bowel disease and possible implications for treatment. *The Lancet Gastroenterology &*

Hepatology, 4(8), 632–642. https://doi.org/10.1016/s2468-1253(19)30089-5

[276] Tomasello, G., Mazzola, M., Leone, A., Sinagra, E., Zummo, G., Farina, F., . . . Cetta, F. (2016). Nutrition, oxidative stress and intestinal dysbiosis: Influence of diet on gut microbiota in inflammatory bowel diseases. *Biomedical Papers of the Faculty of Medicine of Palacký University, Olomouc Czech Republic,* 160(4), 461–466. https://doi.org/10.5507/bp.2016.052

[277] Sugihara, K., & Kamada, N. (2021). Diet–Microbiota interactions in inflammatory bowel disease. *Nutrients,* 13(5), 1533. https://doi.org/10.3390/nu13051533

[278] Allam-Ndoul, B., Castonguay-Paradis, S., & Veilleux, A. (2020). Gut microbiota and intestinal Trans-Epithelial permeability. *International Journal of Molecular Sciences,* 21(17), 6402. https://doi.org/10.3390/ijms21176402

[279] Jackson, D. N., & Theiss, A. L. (2019). Gut bacteria signaling to mitochondria in intestinal inflammation and cancer. *Gut Microbes,* 11(3), 285–304. https://doi.org/10.1080/19490976.2019.1592421

[280] Vancamelbeke, M., & Vermeire, S. (2017b). The intestinal barrier: a fundamental role in health and disease. *Expert Review of Gastroenterology & Hepatology,* 11(9), 821–834. https://doi.org/10.1080/17474124.2017.1343143

[281] Alonso, C., Vicario, M., Pigrau, M., Lobo, B., & Santos, J. (2014). Intestinal barrier function and the Brain-Gut axis. *Advances in Experimental Medicine and Biology* (pp. 73–113). https://doi.org/10.1007/978-1-4939-0897-4_4

[282] Fernández-Tomé, S., Moreno, L., Chaparro, M., & Gisbert, J. P. (2021). Gut microbiota and dietary factors as modulators of the mucus layer in inflammatory bowel disease. *International Journal of Molecular Sciences,* 22(19), 10224. https://doi.org/10.3390/ijms221910224

[283] Birchenough, G., Schroeder, B. O., Bäckhed, F., & Hansson, G. C. (2018). Dietary destabilisation of the balance between the microbiota and the colonic mucus barrier. *Gut Microbes*, 10(2), 246–250. https://doi.org/10.1080/19490976.2018.1513765

[284] Alam, A., & Neish, A. S. (2018). Role of gut microbiota in intestinal wound healing and barrier function. *Tissue Barriers*, 6(3), 1539595. https://doi.org/10.1080/21688370.2018.1539595

[285] Chancharoenthana, W., Kamolratanakul, S., Schultz, M. J., & Leelahavanichkul, A. (2023). The leaky gut and the gut microbiome in sepsis – targets in research and treatment. *Clinical Science*, 137(8), 645–662. https://doi.org/10.1042/cs20220777

[286] Di Vincenzo, F., Del Gaudio, A., Petito, V., Lopetuso, L. R., & Scaldaferri, F. (2023). Gut microbiota, intestinal permeability, and systemic inflammation: a narrative review. *Internal and Emergency Medicine*. https://doi.org/10.1007/s11739-023-03374-w

[287] Johnstone, K. F., & Herzberg, M. C. (2022). Antimicrobial peptides: Defending the mucosal epithelial barrier. *Frontiers in Oral Health*, 3. https://doi.org/10.3389/froh.2022.958480

[288] Venegas, D. P., De La Fuente, M. K., Landskron, G., González, M. J., Quera, R., Dijkstra, G., . . . Hermoso, M. A. (2019). Short chain fatty acids (SCFAs)-Mediated gut epithelial and immune regulation and its relevance for inflammatory bowel diseases. *Frontiers in Immunology,* 10. https://doi.org/10.3389/fimmu.2019.00277

[289] Deleu, S., Machiels, K., Raes, J., Verbeke, K., & Vermeire, S. (2021). Short chain fatty acids and its producing organisms: An overlooked therapy for IBD? *EBioMedicine*, 66, 103293. https://doi.org/10.1016/j.ebiom.2021.103293

[290] Kelly, C., Zheng, L., Campbell, E. L., Saeedi, B., Scholz, C. C., Bayless, A. J., . . . Colgan, S. P. (2015). Crosstalk between Microbiota-Derived Short-Chain Fatty Acids and Intestinal

Epithelial HIF Augments Tissue Barrier Function. *Cell Host & Microbe*, 17(5), 662–671. https://doi.org/10.1016/j.chom.2015.03.005

[291] Gasaly, N., De Vos, P., & Hermoso, M. A. (2021). Impact of bacterial metabolites on gut barrier function and host immunity: A focus on bacterial metabolism and its relevance for intestinal inflammation. *Frontiers in Immunology*, 12. https://doi.org/10.3389/fimmu.2021.658354

[292] Liang, L., Liu, L., Zhou, W., Yang, C., Mai, G., Li, H., & Chen, Y. (2022). Gut microbiota-derived butyrate regulates gut mucus barrier repair by activating the macrophage/WNT/ERK signaling pathway. *Clinical Science*, 136(4), 291–307. https://doi.org/10.1042/cs20210778

[293] Martin-Gallausiaux, C., Marinelli, L., Blottière, H. M., Larraufie, P., & Lapaque, N. (2020). SCFA: mechanisms and functional importance in the gut. *Proceedings of the Nutrition Society*, 80(1), 37–49. https://doi.org/10.1017/s0029665120006916

[294] Fu, Y., Jin, L., & Wang, S. (2023). The role of intestinal microbes on intestinal barrier function and host immunity from a metabolite perspective. *Frontiers in Immunology*, 14, 1277102. https://doi.org/10.3389/fimmu.2023.1277102

[295] Zhang, M., Wang, Y., Zhao, X., Liu, C., Wang, B., & Zha, J. (2021). Mechanistic basis and preliminary practice of butyric acid and butyrate sodium to mitigate gut inflammatory diseases: a comprehensive review. *Nutrition Research*, 95, 1–18. https://doi.org/10.1016/j.nutres.2021.08.007

[296] Brotherton, C., Martin, C., Long, M. D., Kappelman, M. D., & Sandler, R. S. (2016). Avoidance of fiber is associated with greater risk of Crohn's disease flare in a 6-Month period. *Clinical Gastroenterology and Hepatology*, 14(8), 1130–1136. https://doi.org/10.1016/j.cgh.2015.12.029

[297] Takiishi, T., Fénero, C. I. M., & Câmara, N. O. S. (2017). Intestinal barrier and gut microbiota: Shaping our immune responses throughout life. *Tissue Barriers*, 5(4), e1373208. https://doi.org/10.1080/21688370.2017.1373208

[298] Cader, M. Z., & Kaser, A. (2013). Recent advances in inflammatory bowel disease: mucosal immune cells in intestinal inflammation. *Gut*, 62(11), 1653–1664. https://doi.org/10.1136/gutjnl-2012-303955

[299] Nikoopour, E., & Singh, B. (2014). Reciprocity in Microbiome and Immune System Interactions and its Implications in Disease and Health. *Inflammation and Allergy - Drug Targets*, 13(2), 94–104. https://doi.org/10.2174/1871528113666140330201056

[300] Graham, D. B., & Xavier, R. J. (2023). Conditioning of the immune system by the microbiome. *Trends in Immunology*, 44(7), 499–511. https://doi.org/10.1016/j.it.2023.05.002

[301] Chen, L., Ruan, G., Cheng, Y., Yi, A., Chen, D., & Wei, Y. (2023). The role of Th17 cells in inflammatory bowel disease and the research progress. *Frontiers in Immunology*, 13. https://doi.org/10.3389/fimmu.2022.1055914

[302] Yan, J., Luo, M., Chen, Z., & He, B. (2020). The function and role of the TH17/TREG cell balance in inflammatory bowel disease. *Journal of Immunology Research*, 2020, 1–8. https://doi.org/10.1155/2020/8813558

[303] Saéz, Á., Gómez-Bris, R., Herrero-Fernández, B., Mingorance, C., Rius, C., & González-Granado, J. (2021). Innate lymphoid cells in intestinal homeostasis and inflammatory bowel disease. *International Journal of Molecular Sciences*, 22(14), 7618. https://doi.org/10.3390/ijms22147618

[304] Kondělková, K., Vokurková, D., Krejsek, J., Borská, L., Fiala, Z., & Andrýs, C. (2010). Regulatory T cells (Treg) and Their Roles in Immune System with Respect to Immunopathological Disorders. *Acta Medica*, 53(2), 73–77. https://doi.org/10.14712/18059694.2016.63

[305] Calvo-Barreiro, L., Zhang, L., Abdel-Rahman, S. A., Naik, S. P., & Gabr, M. T. (2023). Gut Microbial-Derived metabolites as immune modulators of T helper 17 and regulatory T cells. *International Journal of Molecular Sciences, 24*(2), 1806. https://doi.org/10.3390/ijms24021806

[306] Hosseinkhani, F., Heinken, A., Thiele, I., Lindenburg, P. W., Harms, A. C., & Hankemeier, T. (2021). The contribution of gut bacterial metabolites in the human immune signaling pathway of non-communicable diseases. *Gut Microbes, 13*(1). https://doi.org/10.1080/19490976.2021.1882927

[307] Wang, J., Zhu, N., Su, X., Gao, Y., & Yang, R. (2023). Gut-Microbiota-Derived metabolites maintain gut and systemic immune homeostasis. *Cells, 12*(5), 793. https://doi.org/10.3390/cells12050793

[308] Baxter, N. T., Schmidt, A. W., Venkataraman, A., Kim, K. S., Waldron, C., & Schmidt, T. M. (2019). Dynamics of Human Gut Microbiota and Short-Chain Fatty Acids in Response to Dietary Interventions with Three Fermentable Fibers. *MBio, 10*(1). https://doi.org/10.1128/mbio.02566-18

[309] Arpaia, N., Campbell, C., Fan, X., Dikiy, S., Van Der Veeken, J., deRoos, P., . . . Rudensky, A. Y. (2013). Metabolites produced by commensal bacteria promote peripheral regulatory T-cell generation. *Nature, 504*(7480), 451–455. https://doi.org/10.1038/nature12726

[310] Hodgkinson, K. M., Abbar, F. E., Dobranowski, P. A., Manoogian, J., Butcher, J., Figeys, D., . . . Stintzi, A. (2023). Butyrate's role in human health and the current progress towards its clinical application to treat gastrointestinal disease. *Clinical Nutrition, 42*(2), 61–75. https://doi.org/10.1016/j.clnu.2022.10.024

[311] Hamer, H. M., Jonkers, D., Venema, K., Vanhoutvin, S., Troost, F. J., & Brummer, R. J. (2007). Review article: the role of butyrate on colonic function. *Alimentary Pharmacology & Therapeutics*,

27(2), 104–119. https://doi.org/10.1111/j.1365-2036.2007.03562.x

[312] Hamer, H. M., Jonkers, D., Bast, A., Vanhoutvin, S., Fischer, M. a. J. G., Kodde, A., . . . Brummer, R. J. (2009). Butyrate modulates oxidative stress in the colonic mucosa of healthy humans. *Clinical Nutrition*, 28(1), 88–93. https://doi.org/10.1016/j.clnu.2008.11.002

[313] Scharlau, D., Borowicki, A., Habermann, N., Hofmann, T., Klenow, S., Miene, C., . . . Glei, M. (2009b). Mechanisms of primary cancer prevention by butyrate and other products formed during gut flora-mediated fermentation of dietary fibre. *Mutation Research/Reviews in Mutation Research*, 682(1), 39–53. https://doi.org/10.1016/j.mrrev.2009.04.001

[314] Gasaly, N., Hermoso, M. A., & Gotteland, M. (2021). Butyrate and the Fine-Tuning of Colonic Homeostasis: Implication for Inflammatory Bowel Diseases. *International Journal of Molecular Sciences*, 22(6), 3061. https://doi.org/10.3390/ijms22063061

[315] Hajjar, R., Richard, C., & Santos, M. M. (2021). The role of butyrate in surgical and oncological outcomes in colorectal cancer. *American Journal of Physiology-gastrointestinal and Liver Physiology*, 320(4), G601–G608. https://doi.org/10.1152/ajpgi.00316.2020

[316] Wang, W., Fang, D., Zhang, H., Xue, J., Wangchuk, D., Du, J., & Jiang, L. (2020). <p>Sodium Butyrate Selectively Kills Cancer Cells and Inhibits Migration in Colorectal Cancer by Targeting Thioredoxin-1. *OncoTargets and Therapy*, Volume 13, 4691–4704. https://doi.org/10.2147/ott.s235575

[317] Zhang, J., Yi, M., Zha, L., Chen, S., Li, Z., Li, C., . . . Sun, S. (2016). Sodium butyrate induces endoplasmic reticulum stress and autophagy in colorectal cells: Implications for apoptosis. *PLOS ONE*, 11(1), e0147218. https://doi.org/10.1371/journal.pone.0147218

[318] Levine, A., Rhodes, J. M., Lindsay, J. O., Abreu, M. T., Kamm, M. A., Gibson, P. R., . . . Lewis, J. D. (2020). Dietary guidance from the International Organization for the Study of Inflammatory Bowel Diseases. *Clinical Gastroenterology and Hepatology*, 18(6), 1381–1392. https://doi.org/10.1016/j.cgh.2020.01.046

[319] Dimidi, E., Cox, S., Rossi, M., & Whelan, K. (2019). Fermented foods: definitions and characteristics, impact on the gut microbiota and effects on gastrointestinal health and disease. *Nutrients*, 11(8), 1806. https://doi.org/10.3390/nu11081806

[320] Pace, L., & Crowe, S. E. (2016). Complex relationships between food, diet, and the microbiome. *Gastroenterology Clinics of North America*, 45(2), 253–265. https://doi.org/10.1016/j.gtc.2016.02.004

[321] Ispas, S., Tuță, L., Botnarciuc, M., Ispas, V., Staicovici, S., Ali, S. S., . . . Petcu, A. (2023). Metabolic Disorders, the Microbiome as an Endocrine Organ, and Their Relations with Obesity: A Literature Review. *Journal of Personalized Medicine*, 13(11), 1602. https://doi.org/10.3390/jpm13111602

[322] Reeves, A. R., D'Elia, J., Frías, J., & Salyers, A. A. (1996). A Bacteroides thetaiotaomicron outer membrane protein that is essential for utilization of maltooligosaccharides and starch. *Journal of Bacteriology*, 178(3), 823–830. https://doi.org/10.1128/jb.178.3.823-830.1996

[323] Ndeh, D., Baslé, A., Strahl, H., Yates, E. A., McClurg, U. L., Henrissat, B., . . . Cartmell, A. (2020). Metabolism of multiple glycosaminoglycans by Bacteroides thetaiotaomicron is orchestrated by a versatile core genetic locus. *Nature Communications*, 11(1). https://doi.org/10.1038/s41467-020-14509-4

[324] Kolodziejczyk, A. A., Zheng, D., Shibolet, O., & Elinav, E. (2018). The role of the microbiome in NAFLD and NASH. *EMBO Molecular Medicine*, 11(2). https://doi.org/10.15252/emmm.201809302

[325] Verdier, J., Luedde, T., & Sellge, G. (2015). Biliary mucosal barrier and microbiome. *Visceral Medicine*, 31(3), 156–161. https://doi.org/10.1159/000431071

[326] Carr, T. F., Alkatib, R., & Kraft, M. (2019). Microbiome in mechanisms of asthma. *Clinics in Chest Medicine*, 40(1), 87–96. https://doi.org/10.1016/j.ccm.2018.10.006

[327] Aguilera, A., Dagher, I. A., & Kloepfer, K. M. (2020). Role of the microbiome in allergic disease development. *Current Allergy and Asthma Reports,* 20(9). https://doi.org/10.1007/s11882-020-00944-2

CHAPTER 7. IDENTITY CRISIS: AUTO-IMMUNE DISEASES

[328] Vulcan – mythopedia. (n.d.). Retrieved from https://mythopedia.com/topics/vulcan

[329] Wikipedia contributors. (2023b, December 27). Agni. Retrieved from https://en.wikipedia.org/wiki/Agni

[330] auto- | Etymology of prefix auto- by etymonline. (n.d.). Retrieved from https://www.etymonline.com/word/auto-#etymonline_v_18968

[331] Surace, A. E. A., & Hedrich, C. M. (2019). The role of Epigenetics in Autoimmune/Inflammatory Disease. *Frontiers in Immunology,* 10. https://doi.org/10.3389/fimmu.2019.01525

[332] Jeffries, M. A., & Sawalha, A. H. (2014). Autoimmune disease in the epigenetic era: how has epigenetics changed our understanding of disease and how can we expect the field to evolve? *Expert Review of Clinical Immunology,* 11(1), 45–58. https://doi.org/10.1586/1744666x.2015.994507

[333] Bogdanos, D. P., Smyk, D. S., Rigopoulou, E. I., Mytilinaiou, M., Heneghan, M. A., Selmi, C., & Gershwin, M. E. (2012). Twin studies in autoimmune disease: Genetics, gender and environment. *Journal of Autoimmunity*, 38(2–3), J156–J169. https://doi.org/10.1016/j.jaut.2011.11.003

[334] Ceribelli, A., & Selmi, C. (2020). Epigenetic methods and twin studies. *Advances in Experimental Medicine and Biology* (pp. 95–104). https://doi.org/10.1007/978-981-15-3449-2_3

[335] Leslie, R., & Hawa, M. (1994). Twin studies in auto-immune disease. *Acta Geneticae Medicae Et Gemellologiae*, 43(1–2), 71–81. https://doi.org/10.1017/s000156600000297x

[336] Ingelfinger, F., Gerdes, L. A., Kavaka, V., Krishnarajah, S., Friebel, E., Galli, E., . . . Becher, B. (2022). Twin study reveals non-heritable immune perturbations in multiple sclerosis. *Nature*, 603(7899), 152–158. https://doi.org/10.1038/s41586-022-04419-4

[337] Williams, K. L., Enslow, R., Suresh, S., Beaton, C., Hodge, M., & Brooks, A. E. (2023). Using the microbiome as a regenerative medicine strategy for autoimmune diseases. *Biomedicines*, 11(6), 1582. https://doi.org/10.3390/biomedicines11061582

[338] Hirschberg, S., Gisevius, B., Duscha, A., & Haghikia, A. (2019). Implications of diet and the gut microbiome in neuroinflammatory and neurodegenerative diseases. *International Journal of Molecular Sciences*, 20(12), 3109. https://doi.org/10.3390/ijms20123109

[339] Manzel, A., Müller, D. N., Hafler, D. A., Erdman, S. E., Linker, R., & Kleinewietfeld, M. (2013). Role of "Western diet" in inflammatory autoimmune diseases. *Current Allergy and Asthma Reports*, 14(1). https://doi.org/10.1007/s11882-013-0404-6

[340] Dourado, E., Ferro, M., Guerreiro, C. S., & Fonseca, J. E. (2020). Diet as a modulator of intestinal microbiota in rheumatoid arthritis. *Nutrients*, 12(11), 3504. https://doi.org/10.3390/nu12113504

[341] Petta, I., Fraussen, J., Somers, V., & Kleinewietfeld, M. (2018). Interrelation of diet, gut microbiome, and autoantibody production. *Frontiers in Immunology*, 9, 439 https://doi.org/10.3389/fimmu.2018.00439

[342] Mousa, W. K., Chehadeh, F., & Husband, S. (2022). Microbial dysbiosis in the gut drives systemic autoimmune diseases. *Frontiers in Immunology,* 13. https://doi.org/10.3389/fimmu.2022.906258

[343] Yaigoub, H., Fath, N., Tirichen, H., Wu, C., Li, R., & Li, Y. (2022). Bidirectional crosstalk between dysbiotic gut microbiota and systemic lupus erythematosus: What is new in therapeutic approaches? *Clinical Immunology,* 244, 109109. https://doi.org/10.1016/j.clim.2022.109109

[344] Marietta, E., Horwath, I., Balakrishnan, B., & Taneja, V. (2019). Role of the intestinal microbiome in autoimmune diseases and its use in treatments. *Cellular Immunology,* 339, 50–58. https://doi.org/10.1016/j.cellimm.2018.10.005

[345] Han, H., Li, Y., Fang, J., Liu, G., Yin, J., Li, T., & Yin, Y. (2018). Gut microbiota and type 1 diabetes. *International Journal of Molecular Sciences,* 19(4), 995. https://doi.org/10.3390/ijms19040995

[346] Fu, X., Chen, Y., & Chen, D. (2020). The role of gut microbiome in autoimmune uveitis. *Ophthalmic Research,* 64(2), 168–177. https://doi.org/10.1159/000510212

[347] Engels, N., & Wienands, J. (2018). Memory control by the B cell antigen receptor. *Immunological Reviews,* 283(1), 150–160. https://doi.org/10.1111/imr.12651

[348] Pennock, N. D., White, J. T., Cross, E. W., Cheney, E. E., Tamburini, B., & Kedl, R. M. (2013). T cell responses: naïve to memory and everything in between. *Advances in Physiology Education,* 37(4), 273–283. https://doi.org/10.1152/advan.00066.2013

[349] Rojas, M., Restrepo-Jiménez, P., Monsalve, D. M., Pacheco, Y., Acosta-Ampudia, Y., Ramírez-Santana, C., . . . Anaya, J. (2018). Molecular mimicry and autoimmunity. *Journal of Autoimmunity,* 95, 100–123. https://doi.org/10.1016/j.jaut.2018.10.012

[350] Albert, L., & Inman, R. D. (1999). Molecular Mimicry and Autoimmunity. *The New England Journal of Medicine*, 341(27), 2068–2074. https://doi.org/10.1056/nejm199912303412707

[351] Vojdani, A. (2015). Molecular mimicry as a mechanism for food immune reactivities and autoimmunity. *Alternative therapies in health and medicine*, 21 Suppl 1, 34–45. Retrieved from https://pubmed.ncbi.nlm.nih.gov/25599184

[352] Vojdani, A., Gushgari, L. R., & Vojdani, E. (2020). Interaction between food antigens and the immune system: Association with autoimmune disorders. *Autoimmunity Reviews*, 19(3), 102459. https://doi.org/10.1016/j.autrev.2020.102459

[353] Wildner, G., & Diedrichs-Möhring, M. (2020). Molecular mimicry and uveitis. *Frontiers in Immunology*, 11. https://doi.org/10.3389/fimmu.2020.580636

[354] Vaarala, O. (2011). The gut as a regulator of early inflammation in type 1 diabetes. *Current Opinion in Endocrinology, Diabetes and Obesity,* 18(4), 241–247. https://doi.org/10.1097/med.0b013e3283488218

[355] Lamb, M. M., Miller, M. R., Seifert, J., Frederiksen, B. N., Kroehl, M., Rewers, M., & Norris, J. M. (2014). The effect of childhood cow's milk intake and HLA-DR genotype on risk of islet autoimmunity and type 1 diabetes: The Diabetes Autoimmunity Study in the Young. *Pediatric Diabetes*, 16(1), 31–38. https://doi.org/10.1111/pedi.12115

[356] Saukkonen, T., Virtanen, S. M., Karppinen, M., Reijonen, H., Ilonen, J., Räsänen, L., . . . Savilahti, E. (1998). Significance of cow's milk protein antibodies as risk factor for childhood IDDM: interactions with dietary cow's milk intake and HLA-DQB1 genotype. *Diabetologia*, 41(1), 72–78. https://doi.org/10.1007/s001250050869

[357] Lampousi, A., Carlsson, S., & Löfvenborg, J. E. (2021). Dietary factors and risk of islet autoimmunity and type 1 diabetes: a

systematic review and meta-analysis. *EBioMedicine*, 72, 103633. https://doi.org/10.1016/j.ebiom.2021.103633

[358] Benslama, Y., Dennouni-Medjati, N., Dali-Sahi, M., Meziane, F. Z., & Harek, Y. (2021). Childhood type 1 diabetes mellitus and risk factor of interactions between dietary cow's milk intake and HLA-DR3/DR4 genotype. *Journal of Biomolecular Structure & Dynamics*, 40(21), 10931–10939. https://doi.org/10.1080/07391102.2021.1953599

[359] Lempainen, J., Tauriainen, S., Vaarala, O., Mäkelä, M., Honkanen, H., Marttila, J., . . . Ilonen, J. (2012). Interaction of enterovirus infection and cow's milk-based formula nutrition in type 1 diabetes-associated autoimmunity. *Diabetes/Metabolism Research and Reviews*, 28(2), 177–185. https://doi.org/10.1002/dmrr.1294

[360] Virtanen, S. M., Hyppönen, E., Läärä, E., Vähäsalo, P., Kulmala, P., Savola, K., . . . Akerblom, H. K. (1998). Cow's milk consumption, disease-associated autoantibodies and type 1 diabetes mellitus: a follow-up study in siblings of diabetic children. Childhood Diabetes in Finland Study Group. *Diabetic Medicine: A Journal of the British Diabetic Association*, 15(9), 730–738. Retrieved from https://pubmed.ncbi.nlm.nih.gov/9737801/

[361] Dang, M., Buzzetti, R., & Pozzilli, P. (2013). Epigenetics in autoimmune diseases with focus on type 1 diabetes. *Diabetes/Metabolism Research and Reviews*, 29(1), 8–18. https://doi.org/10.1002/dmrr.2375

[362] Monetini, L., Cavallo, M. G., Manfrini, S., Stefanini, L., Picarelli, A., Di Tola, M., . . . Pozzilli, P. (2002). Antibodies to bovine Beta-Casein in diabetes and other autoimmune diseases. *Hormone and Metabolic Research*, 34(8), 455–459. https://doi.org/10.1055/s-2002-33595

[363] Vandenplas, Y., Castrellón, P. G., Rivas, R., Gutiérrez, C. J., Garcia, L. D., Jimenez, J. E., . . . De Alarcón, P. A. (2014). Safety of

soya-based infant formulas in children. *British Journal of Nutrition*, 111(8), 1340–1360. https://doi.org/10.1017/s0007114513003942

[364] Knip, M., Virtanen, S. M., Seppä, K., Ilonen, J., Savilahti, E., Vaarala, O., . . . Åkerblom, H. K. (2010b). Dietary intervention in infancy and later signs of Beta-Cell autoimmunity. *The New England Journal of Medicine*, 363(20), 1900–1908. https://doi.org/10.1056/nejmoa1004809

[365] W, B., Senior, Anderson, G. A., Morley, K. D., & Kerr, M. A. (1999). Evidence that patients with rheumatoid arthritis have asymptomatic 'non-significant' Proteus mirabilis bacteriuria more frequently than healthy controls. *Journal of Infection*, 38(2), 99–106. https://doi.org/10.1016/s0163-4453(99)90076-2

[366] Ebringer, A. (2005). Rheumatoid arthritis and Proteus. *Clinical Medicine*, 5(4), 420.2-421. https://doi.org/10.7861/clinmedicine.5-4-420a

[367] Wilson, C., Thakore, A., Isenberg, D., & Ebringer, A. (1997). Correlation between anti-Proteus antibodies and isolation rates ofP. mirabilis in rheumatoid arthritis. *Rheumatology International*, 16(5), 187–189. https://doi.org/10.1007/bf01330294

[368] Wilson, C., Tiwana, H., & Ebringer, A. (2000). Molecular mimicry between HLA-DR alleles associated with rheumatoid arthritis and Proteus mirabilis as the aetiological basis for autoimmunity. *Microbes and Infection*, 2(12), 1489–1496. https://doi.org/10.1016/s1286-4579(00)01303-4

[369] Ebringer, A., & Rashid, T. (2006). Rheumatoid Arthritis is an Autoimmune Disease Triggered by Proteus Urinary Tract Infection. *Clinical & Developmental Immunology*, 13(1), 41–48. https://doi.org/10.1080/17402520600576578

[370] Rashid, T., & Ebringer, A. (2007). Rheumatoid arthritis is linked to Proteus—the evidence. *Clinical Rheumatology*, 26(7), 1036–1043. https://doi.org/10.1007/s10067-006-0491-z

[371] Luo, Y., Tong, Y., Wu, L., Niu, H., Li, Y., Su, L., . . . Liu, Y. (2023). Alteration of gut microbiota in individuals at High-Risk for rheumatoid arthritis associated with disturbed metabolome and the initiation of arthritis through the triggering of mucosal immunity imbalance. *Arthritis & Rheumatology*, 75(10), 1736–1748. https://doi.org/10.1002/art.42616

[372] Chimenti, M. S., Triggianese, P., Nuccetelli, M., Terracciano, C., Crisanti, A., Guarino, M. D., . . . Perricone, R. (2015). Auto-reactions, autoimmunity and psoriatic arthritis. *Autoimmunity Reviews*, 14(12), 1142–1146. https://doi.org/10.1016/j.autrev.2015.08.003

[373] Kjeldsen-Kragh, J., Rashid, T., Dybwad, A., Sioud, M., Haugen, M., Førre, Ø., & Ebringer, A. (1995). Decrease in anti-Proteus mirabilis but not anti-Escherichia coli antibody levels in rheumatoid arthritis patients treated with fasting and a one year vegetarian diet. *Annals of the Rheumatic Diseases*, 54(3), 221–224. https://doi.org/10.1136/ard.54.3.221

[374] Alwarith, J., Kahleová, H., Rembert, E., Yonas, W. N., Dort, S., Calcagno, M., . . . Barnard, N. D. (2019). Nutrition Interventions in rheumatoid arthritis: The Potential Use of Plant-Based Diets. a review. *Frontiers in Nutrition*, 6. https://doi.org/10.3389/fnut.2019.00141

[375] Bayır, A. G., Mendes, B. P. B., & Dadak, A. (2023). The integral role of diets including natural products to manage rheumatoid arthritis: A Narrative review. *Current Issues in Molecular Biology*, 45(7), 5373–5388. https://doi.org/10.3390/cimb45070341

[376] Peltonen, R., Nenonen, M., Helve, T., Hänninen, O., Toivanen, P., & Eerola, E. (1997). Faecal microbial flora and disease activity in rheumatoid arthritis during a vegan diet. *Rheumatology*, 36(1), 64–68. https://doi.org/10.1093/rheumatology/36.1.64

[377] Karakasis, P., Patoulias, D., Stachteas, P., Lefkou, E., Dimitroulas, T., & Fragakis, N. (2023). Accelerated atherosclerosis and Management of cardiovascular risk in

autoimmune rheumatic diseases: an updated review. *Current Problems in Cardiology*, 48(12), 101999. https://doi.org/10.1016/j.cpcardiol.2023.101999

[378] Funada, S., Luo, Y., Nishioka, N., & Yoshioka, T. (2023). Cardiovascular risk in systemic autoimmune diseases. *The Lancet*, 401(10370), 21. https://doi.org/10.1016/s0140-6736(22)02474-6

[379] Conrad, N., Verbeke, G., Molenberghs, G., Goetschalckx, L., Callender, T., Cambridge, G., . . . Verbakel, J. Y. (2022). Autoimmune diseases and cardiovascular risk: a population-based study on 19 autoimmune diseases and 12 cardiovascular diseases in 22 million individuals in the UK. *The Lancet*, 400(10354), 733–743. https://doi.org/10.1016/s0140-6736(22)01349-6

[380] Jiang, Q., Yang, G., Liu, Q., Wang, S., & Cui, D. (2021). Function and role of regulatory T cells in rheumatoid arthritis. *Frontiers in Immunology*, 12. https://doi.org/10.3389/fimmu.2021.626193

[381] Häger, J., Bang, H., Hagen, M., Frech, M., Träger, P., Sokolova, M. V., . . . Zaiss, M. M. (2019). The role of dietary fiber in rheumatoid arthritis patients: A feasibility study. *Nutrients*, 11(10), 2392. https://doi.org/10.3390/nu11102392

[382] Xu, X., Wang, M., Wang, Z., Chen, Q., Chen, X., Xu, Y., . . . Li, Y. (2022). The bridge of the gut–joint axis: Gut microbial metabolites in rheumatoid arthritis. *Frontiers in Immunology*, 13. https://doi.org/10.3389/fimmu.2022.1007610

[383] Stoiloudis, P., Kesidou, E., Bakirtzis, C., Sintila, S., Konstantinidou, N., Boziki, M., & Grigoriadis, N. (2022). The Role of Diet and Interventions on Multiple Sclerosis: A review. *Nutrients*, 14(6), 1150. https://doi.org/10.3390/nu14061150

[384] Muraven, M., & Baumeister, R. F. (2000). Self-regulation and depletion of limited resources: Does self-control resemble a muscle? *Psychological Bulletin*, 126(2), 247–259. https://doi.org/10.1037/0033-2909.126.2.247

[385] Muraven, M., Shmueli, D., & Burkley, E. (2006). Conserving self-control strength. *Journal of Personality and Social Psychology*, 91(3), 524–537. https://doi.org/10.1037/0022-3514.91.3.524

[386] Tice, D. M., Baumeister, R. F., Shmueli, D., & Muraven, M. (2007). Restoring the self: Positive affect helps improve self-regulation following ego depletion. *Journal of Experimental Social Psychology*, 43(3), 379–384. https://doi.org/10.1016/j.jesp.2006.05.007

CHAPTER 8. WORKING FRAME: JOINTS, BONES, AND MUSCLES.

[387] Martial, Epigrammata, book 5, XXIV. (n.d.). Retrieved from https://www.perseus.tufts.edu/hopper/text?doc=Perseus%3Atext%3A2008.01.0506%3Abook%3D5%3Apoem%3D24

[388] Chisari, E., Wouthuyzen-Bakker, M., Friedrich, A., & Parvizi, J. (2021). The relation between the gut microbiome and osteoarthritis: A systematic review of literature. *PLOS ONE*, 16(12), e0261353. https://doi.org/10.1371/journal.pone.0261353

[389] Guido, G., Ausenda, G., Iascone, V., & Chisari, E. (2021). Gut permeability and osteoarthritis, towards a mechanistic understanding of the pathogenesis: a systematic review. *Annals of Medicine*, 53(1), 2380–2390. https://doi.org/10.1080/07853890.2021.2014557

[390] Hao, X., Shang, X., Liu, J., Chi, R., Zhang, J., & Xu, T. (2021). The gut microbiota in osteoarthritis: where do we stand and what can we do? *Arthritis Research & Therapy*, 23(1). https://doi.org/10.1186/s13075-021-02427-9

[391] Biver, E., Bérenbaum, F., Valdes, A., De Carvalho, I. A., Bindels, L. B., Brandi, M. L., . . . Rizzoli, R. (2019). Gut microbiota and osteoarthritis management: An expert consensus of the European society for clinical and economic aspects of

osteoporosis, osteoarthritis and musculoskeletal diseases (ESCEO). *Ageing Research Reviews*, 55, 100946. https://doi.org/10.1016/j.arr.2019.100946

[392] Park, J. Y., Pillinger, M. H., & Abramson, S. B. (2006). Prostaglandin E2 synthesis and secretion: The role of PGE2 synthases. *Clinical Immunology*, 119(3), 229–240. https://doi.org/10.1016/j.clim.2006.01.016

[393] Calder, P. C. (2007). Dietary arachidonic acid: harmful, harmless or helpful? *British Journal of Nutrition*, 98(3), 451–453. https://doi.org/10.1017/s0007114507761779

[394] Adam, O., Beringer, C., Kless, T., Lemmen, C., Adam, A., Wiseman, M., . . . Förth, W. (2003). Anti-inflammatory effects of a low arachidonic acid diet and fish oil in patients with rheumatoid arthritis. *Rheumatology International*, 23(1), 27–36. https://doi.org/10.1007/s00296-002-0234-7

[395] Clinton, C., O'Brien, S., Law, J., Renier, C. M., & Wendt, M. R. (2015). Whole-Foods, Plant-Based diet alleviates the symptoms of osteoarthritis. *Arthritis*, 2015, 1–9. https://doi.org/10.1155/2015/708152

[396] Caroff, M., & Karibian, D. (2003). Structure of bacterial lipopolysaccharides. *Carbohydrate Research*, 338(23), 2431–2447. https://doi.org/10.1016/j.carres.2003.07.010

[397] Worboys, M. (2017). *The history of surgical wound infection: revolution or evolution?* In Palgrave Macmillan UK eBooks (pp. 215–233). https://doi.org/10.1057/978-1-349-95260-1_11

[398] Lax, A. J. (2005). *The golden age of microbiology*. In Oxford University Press eBooks (pp. 34–63). https://doi.org/10.1093/oso/9780198605584.003.0003

[399] Rietschel, E., & Cavaillon, J. (2003). Richard Pfeiffer and Alexandre Besredka: creators of the concept of endotoxin and anti-endotoxin. *Microbes and Infection*, 5(15), 1407–1414. https://doi.org/10.1016/j.micinf.2003.10.003

[400] Westphal, O., Lüderitz, O., Galanos, C., Mayer, H., & Rietschel, E. (1986). The story of bacterial endotoxin. *Elsevier eBooks* (pp. 13–34). https://doi.org/10.1016/b978-0-08-032008-3.50005-9

[401] Huang, Z., & Kraus, V. B. (2015). Does lipopolysaccharide-mediated inflammation have a role in OA? *Nature Reviews Rheumatology,* 12(2), 123–129. https://doi.org/10.1038/nrrheum.2015.158

[402] Silvestre, M. P., Rodrigues, A. M., Marques, C., Teixeira, D., Calhau, C., & Branco, J. (2020). Cross-Talk between Diet-Associated Dysbiosis and Hand Osteoarthritis. *Nutrients*, 12(11), 3469. https://doi.org/10.3390/nu12113469

[403] Erlanson-Albertsson, C., & Stenkula, K. G. (2021). The importance of food for endotoxemia and an inflammatory response. *International Journal of Molecular Sciences*, 22(17), 9562. https://doi.org/10.3390/ijms22179562

[404] Quintanilha, B. J., Ferreira, L. R. P., Ferreira, F. M., Cunha-Neto, E., Sampaio, G. R., & Rogero, M. M. (2020). Circulating plasma microRNAs dysregulation and metabolic endotoxemia induced by a high-fat high-saturated diet. *Clinical Nutrition*, 39(2), 554–562. https://doi.org/10.1016/j.clnu.2019.02.042

[405] Mohammad, S., & Thiemermann, C. (2021). Role of metabolic endotoxemia in systemic inflammation and potential interventions. *Frontiers in Immunology*, 11.594150. https://doi.org/10.3389/fimmu.2020.594150

[406] Castro-Barquero, S., Casas, R., Rimm, E. B., Tresserra-Rimbau, A., Romaguera, D., Martínéz, J. A., . . . Estruch, R. (2023). Loss of Visceral Fat is Associated with a Reduction in Inflammatory Status in Patients with Metabolic Syndrome. *Molecular Nutrition & Food Research*, 67(4). https://doi.org/10.1002/mnfr.202200264

[407] Zhang, K., Wang, L., Liu, Z., Geng, B., Teng, Y., Liu, X., . . . Xia, Y. (2021). Mechanosensory and mechanotransductive processes mediated by ion channels in articular chondrocytes: Potential

therapeutic targets for osteoarthritis. *Channels,* 15(1), 339–359. https://doi.org/10.1080/19336950.2021.1903184
[408] Felson, D. T. (1996b). Weight and osteoarthritis. *The American Journal of Clinical Nutrition,* 63(3), 430S-432S. https://doi.org/10.1093/ajcn/63.3.430
[409] Wikipedia contributors. (2023, December 22). Kubera. Retrieved from https://en.wikipedia.org/wiki/Kubera
[410] Dhurandhar, E. J. (2016). The food-insecurity obesity paradox: A resource scarcity hypothesis. *Physiology & Behavior,* 162, 88–92. https://doi.org/10.1016/j.physbeh.2016.04.025
[411] Ranjit, N., Macias, S., & Hoelscher, D. M. (2020). Factors related to poor diet quality in food insecure populations. *Translational Behavioral Medicine,* 10(6), 1297–1305. https://doi.org/10.1093/tbm/ibaa028
[412] evel, M., Tsai, M., Parham, A., Andrzejak, S. E., Jones, S. R., & Moore, J. X. (2023). Association of food deserts and food swamps with Obesity-Related cancer mortality in the US. *JAMA Oncology,* 9(7), 909. https://doi.org/10.1001/jamaoncol.2023.0634
[413] Palacios, C. (2006). The Role of Nutrients in Bone Health, from A to Z. *Critical Reviews in Food Science and Nutrition,* 46(8), 621–628. https://doi.org/10.1080/10408390500466174
[414] Kitchin, B., & Morgan, S. (2007). Not just calcium and vitamin D: Other nutritional considerations in osteoporosis. *Current Rheumatology Reports,* 9(1), 85–92. https://doi.org/10.1007/s11926-007-0027-9
[415] Groenendijk, I., Van Delft, M., Versloot, P., Van Loon, L. J., & De Groot, L. C. P. G. M. (2022). Impact of magnesium on bone health in older adults: A systematic review and meta-analysis. *Bone,* 154, 116233. https://doi.org/10.1016/j.bone.2021.116233
[416] Office of Dietary Supplements - Vitamin K. (n.d.). Retrieved from https://ods.od.nih.gov/factsheets/vitaminK-HealthProfessional/#h3

[417] Office of Dietary Supplements - magnesium. (n.d.). Retrieved from https://ods.od.nih.gov/factsheets/Magnesium-Consumer/#h3

[418] Scialla, J. J., & Anderson, C. A. (2013). Dietary acid load: a novel nutritional target in chronic kidney disease? *Advances in Chronic Kidney Disease*, 20(2), 141–149. https://doi.org/10.1053/j.ackd.2012.11.001

[419] Breslau, N. A., Brinkley, L., Hill, K., & Pak, C. Y. (1988). Relationship of animal Protein-Rich diet to kidney stone formation and calcium metabolism*. *The Journal of Clinical Endocrinology & Metabolism*, 66(1), 140–146. https://doi.org/10.1210/jcem-66-1-140

[420] D'Alessandro, C., Ferraro, P. M., Cianchi, C., Barsotti, M., Gambaro, G., & Cupisti, A. (2019). Which diet for Calcium Stone Patients: A Real-World Approach to Preventive Care. *Nutrients*, 11(5), 1182. https://doi.org/10.3390/nu11051182

[421] Thorpe, M., & Evans, E. M. (2011). Dietary protein and bone health: harmonizing conflicting theories. *Nutrition Reviews*, 69(4), 215–230. https://doi.org/10.1111/j.1753-4887.2011.00379.x

[422] Tsagari, A. (2020). Dietary protein intake and bone health. *Journal of Frailty, Sarcopenia and Falls*, 05(01), 1–5. https://doi.org/10.22540/jfsf-05-001

[423] Manolagas, S. C. (2010). From Estrogen-Centric to aging and Oxidative Stress: A Revised perspective of the Pathogenesis of Osteoporosis. *Endocrine Reviews*, 31(3), 266–300. https://doi.org/10.1210/er.2009-0024

[424] Mohamad, N., Ima-Nirwana, S., & Chin, K. (2020). Are oxidative stress and inflammation mediators of bone loss due to estrogen deficiency? A review of current evidence. *Endocrine, Metabolic & Immune Disorders*, 20(9), 1478–1487. https://doi.org/10.2174/1871530320666200604160614

[425] Pellegrino, A., Tiidus, P. M., & Vandenboom, R. (2022). Mechanisms of estrogen influence on skeletal muscle: mass, regeneration, and mitochondrial function. *Sports Medicine*, 52(12), 2853–2869. https://doi.org/10.1007/s40279-022-01733-9

[426] Golbidi, S., Li, H., & Laher, I. (2018). Oxidative stress: a unifying mechanism for cell damage induced by noise, (Water-Pipe) smoking, and emotional Stress—Therapeutic Strategies Targeting redox imbalance. *Antioxidants & Redox Signaling*, 28(9), 741–759. https://doi.org/10.1089/ars.2017.7257

[427] Münzel, T., & Daiber, A. (2018). Environmental Stressors and Their Impact on Health and Disease with Focus on Oxidative Stress. *Antioxidants & Redox Signaling*, 28(9), 735–740. https://doi.org/10.1089/ars.2017.7488

[428] Bloomfield S. A. (2001). Cellular and molecular mechanisms for the bone response to mechanical loading. *International journal of sport nutrition and exercise metabolism*, 11 Suppl, S128–S136. https://doi.org/10.1123/ijsnem.11.s1.s128

[429] Warden, S. J., Sventeckis, A. M., Surowiec, R. K., & Fuchs, R. K. (2022). Enhanced Bone Size, Microarchitecture, and Strength in Female Runners with a History of Playing Multidirectional Sports. *Medicine and Science in Sports and Exercise*, 54(12), 2020–2030. https://doi.org/10.1249/mss.0000000000003016

[430] Clissold, T. L., Cronin, J., De Souza, M. J., Wilson, D. R., & Winwood, P. (2020). Bilateral multidirectional jumps with reactive jump-landings achieve osteogenic thresholds with and without instruction in premenopausal women. *Clinical Biomechanics*, 73, 1–8. https://doi.org/10.1016/j.clinbiomech.2019.12.025

[431] Tucker, L. A., Strong, J. E., LeCheminant, J. D., & Bailey, B. W. (2015). Effect of two jumping programs on hip bone mineral density in premenopausal women: a randomized controlled trial.

American Journal of Health Promotion, 29(3), 158–164. https://doi.org/10.4278/ajhp.130430-quan-200

[432] Wikipedia contributors. (2024, January 4). Bharatanatyam. Retrieved from https://en.wikipedia.org/wiki/Bharatanatyam

[433] Teegarden, D., Proulx, W. R., Martin, B. R., Zhao, J., McCabe, G. P., Lyle, R. M., . . . Weaver, C. M. (1995). Peak bone mass in young women. *Journal of Bone and Mineral Research*, 10(5), 711–715. https://doi.org/10.1002/jbmr.5650100507

[434] Naderi, A., Gobbi, N., Ali, A., Berjisian, E., Hamidvand, A., Forbes, S. C., . . . Saunders, B. (2023). Carbohydrates and Endurance Exercise: A Narrative review of a food first approach. *Nutrients*, 15(6), 1367. https://doi.org/10.3390/nu15061367

[435] Harvard Health Publishing. Time for more Vitamin D. https://www.health.harvard.edu/staying-healthy/time-for-more-vitamin-d Accessed on 01/07/2024.

[436] Webb, A. R., & Engelsen, O. (2020). Ultraviolet exposure scenarios: balancing risks of erythema and benefits of cutaneous vitamin D synthesis. *Advances in Experimental Medicine and Biology* (pp. 387–405). https://doi.org/10.1007/978-3-030-46227-7_20

[437] Walston, J. D. (2012). Sarcopenia in older adults. *Current Opinion in Rheumatology*, 24(6), 623–627. https://doi.org/10.1097/bor.0b013e328358d59b

[438] Coll, P. P., Phu, S., Hajjar, S. H., Kirk, B., Duque, G., & Taxel, P. (2021). The prevention of osteoporosis and sarcopenia in older adults. *Journal of the American Geriatrics Society*, 69(5), 1388–1398. https://doi.org/10.1111/jgs.17043

[439] Laviano, A., Gori, C., & Rianda, S. (2014). Sarcopenia and nutrition. *Advances in food and nutrition research* (pp. 101–136). https://doi.org/10.1016/b978-0-12-800270-4.00003-1

[440] Abiri, B., & Vafa, M. (2017). Nutrition and sarcopenia: A review of the evidence of nutritional influences. *Critical Reviews*

in *Food Science and Nutrition*, 59(9), 1456–1466. https://doi.org/10.1080/10408398.2017.1412940

[441] Anton, S. D., Hida, A., Mankowski, R. T., Layne, A. S., Solberg, L. M., Mainous, A. G., & Buford, T. W. (2018). *Nutrition and exercise in Sarcopenia. Current Protein & Peptide Science*, 19(7), 649–667. https://doi.org/10.2174/1389203717666161227144349

[442] Colón, C. J. P., Collado, P. S., & Cuevas, M. J. (2014). [Benefits of strength training for the prevention and treatment of sarcopenia]. *DOAJ (DOAJ: Directory of Open Access Journals)*, 29(5), 979–988. https://doi.org/10.3305/nh.2014.29.5.7313

[443] Robinson, S., Granic, A., & Sayer, A. A. (2019). Nutrition and muscle strength, as the key component of sarcopenia: An overview of current evidence. *Nutrients*, 11(12), 2942. https://doi.org/10.3390/nu11122942

[444] Du, Y., Oh, C., & No, J. (2018). Associations between Sarcopenia and Metabolic Risk Factors: A Systematic Review and Meta-Analysis. *Journal of Obesity & Metabolic Syndrome*, 27(3), 175–185. https://doi.org/10.7570/jomes.2018.27.3.175

[445] Kreouzi, M., Theodorakis, N., & Constantinou, C. (2022). Lessons Learned from Blue Zones, Lifestyle Medicine Pillars and Beyond: An update on the contributions of behavior and genetics to wellbeing and longevity. *American Journal of Lifestyle Medicine,* 155982762211184. https://doi.org/10.1177/15598276221118494

[446] Herbert, C., House, M., Dietzman, R., Climstein, M., Furness, J., & Kemp-Smith, K. (2022). Blue Zones: Centenarian Modes of Physical Activity: A scoping review. *Journal of Population Ageing*. https://doi.org/10.1007/s12062-022-09396-0

[447] Denison, H., Cooper, C., Sayer, A. A., & Robinson, S. (2015). Prevention and optimal management of sarcopenia: a review of combined exercise and nutrition interventions to improve

muscle outcomes in older people. *Clinical Interventions in Aging*, 859. https://doi.org/10.2147/cia.s55842

[448] Buettner, D. (2023, January 9). Blue Zones Diet: Food Secrets of the World's Longest-Lived People. Retrieved from https://www.bluezones.com/2020/07/blue-zones-diet-food-secrets-of-the-worlds-longest-lived-people/ Accessed on 01/07/2024

[449] Zamboni, M., Mazzali, G., Fantin, F., Rossi, A. P., & Di Francesco, V. (2008). Sarcopenic obesity: A new category of obesity in the elderly. *Nutrition, Metabolism and Cardiovascular Diseases*, 18(5), 388–395. https://doi.org/10.1016/j.numecd.2007.10.002

[450] Maheshwari, V., & Basu, S. (2023). Sarcopenic obesity Burden, determinants, and association with risk of frailty, falls, and functional impairment in older adults with diabetes: A Propensity Score Matching analysis. *Cureus.15*(11), e49601. https://doi.org/10.7759/cureus.49601

[451] Rolland, Y., Lauwers-Cancès, V., Cristini, C., Van Kan, G. A., Janssen, I., Morley, J. E., & Vellas, B. (2009). Difficulties with physical function associated with obesity, sarcopenia, and sarcopenic-obesity in community-dwelling elderly women: the EPIDOS (EPIDemiologie de l'OSteoporose) Study. *The American Journal of Clinical Nutrition,* 89(6), 1895–1900. https://doi.org/10.3945/ajcn.2008.26950

[452] Lösch, S., Moghaddam, N., Großschmidt, K., Risser, D., & Kanz, F. (2014). Stable Isotope and Trace Element Studies on Gladiators and Contemporary Romans from Ephesus (Turkey, 2nd and 3rd Ct. AD) - Implications for Differences in Diet. *PLOS ONE*, 9(10), e110489. https://doi.org/10.1371/journal.pone.0110489

[453] Mason, P. (2014). Roman gladiators knew the value of calcium. *The Pharmaceutical Journal*, 293. Retrieved from

https://pharmaceutical-journal.com/article/opinion/roman-gladiators-knew-the-value-of-calcium

CHAPTER 9. MEMORY SAVINGS FOR THE FUTURE: BRAIN HEALTH

[454] Santonastaso, O., Zaccari, V., Crescentini, C., Fabbro, F., Capurso, V., Vicari, S., & Menghini, D. (2020). Clinical Application of Mindfulness-Oriented Meditation: A Preliminary Study in Children with ADHD. *International Journal of Environmental Research and Public Health*, 17(18), 6916. https://doi.org/10.3390/ijerph17186916

[455] Poissant, H., Mendrek, A., Talbot, N., Khoury, B., & Nolan, J. A. (2019). Behavioral and Cognitive Impacts of Mindfulness-Based Interventions on Adults with Attention-Deficit Hyperactivity Disorder: *A Systematic Review. Behavioural Neurology*, 2019, 1–16. https://doi.org/10.1155/2019/5682050

[456] Mitchell, J. T., McIntyre, E., English, J. S., Dennis, M. F., Beckham, J. C., & Kollins, S. H. (2013). A pilot trial of mindfulness meditation training for ADHD in Adulthood: impact on core symptoms, executive functioning, and emotion dysregulation. *Journal of Attention Disorders*, 21(13), 1105–1120. https://doi.org/10.1177/1087054713513328

[457] Basso, J. C., McHale, A. L., Ende, V., Oberlin, D. J., & Suzuki, W. (2019). Brief, daily meditation enhances attention, memory, mood, and emotional regulation in non-experienced meditators. *Behavioural Brain Research*, 356, 208–220. https://doi.org/10.1016/j.bbr.2018.08.023

[458] Prakash, R. S. (2021). Mindfulness meditation: Impact on attentional control and emotion dysregulation. *Archives of clinical neuropsychology : the official journal of the National Academy of Neuropsychologists*, 36(7), 1283–1290. https://doi.org/10.1093/arclin/acab053

[459] Evans, S., Ling, M., Hill, B., Rinehart, N., Austin, D. W., & Sciberras, E. (2017). Systematic review of meditation-based interventions for children with ADHD. *European Child & Adolescent Psychiatry*, 27(1), 9–27. https://doi.org/10.1007/s00787-017-1008-9

[460] Whitfield, T., Barnhofer, T., Acabchuk, R. L., Cohen, A., Lee, M., Schlosser, M., . . . Marchant, N. L. (2021). The Effect of mindfulness-based programs on Cognitive Function in Adults: A systematic review and meta-analysis. *Neuropsychology Review*, 32(3), 677–702. https://doi.org/10.1007/s11065-021-09519-y

[461] Gard, T., Hölzel, B. K., & Lazar, S. W. (2014). The potential effects of meditation on age-related cognitive decline: a systematic review. *Annals of the New York Academy of Sciences*, 1307(1), 89–103. https://doi.org/10.1111/nyas.12348

[462] Gill, L., Renault, R., Campbell, E., Rainville, P., & Khoury, B. (2020). Mindfulness induction and cognition: A systematic review and meta-analysis. *Consciousness and Cognition*, 84, 102991. https://doi.org/10.1016/j.concog.2020.102991

[463] Mirabito, G., & Verhaeghen, P. (2022). The Effects of mindfulness interventions on Older Adults' Cognition: A Meta-Analysis. *The Journals of Gerontology: Series B*, 78(3), 394–408. https://doi.org/10.1093/geronb/gbac143

[464] Farhang, M., Miranda-Castillo, C., Rubio, M., & Furtado, G. E. (2019). Impact of mind-body interventions in older adults with mild cognitive impairment: a systematic review. *International Psychogeriatrics*, 31(5), 643–666. https://doi.org/10.1017/s1041610218002302

[465] Bulzacka, E., Lavault, S., Pélissolo, A., & Isnard, C. (2018). Mindful neuropsychology : repenser la réhabilitation neuropsychologique à travers la pleine conscience. *L'Encéphale*, 44(1), 75–82. https://doi.org/10.1016/j.encep.2017.03.006

[466] Chiesa, A., Calati, R., & Serretti, A. (2011). Does mindfulness training improve cognitive abilities? A systematic review of

neuropsychological findings. *Clinical Psychology Review*, 31(3), 449–464. https://doi.org/10.1016/j.cpr.2010.11.003

[467] National Institute on Aging. (n.d.-b). Do's and Don'ts: Communicating With a Person Who Has Alzheimer's Disease. Retrieved January 8, 2024, from https://www.nia.nih.gov/health/alzheimers-changes-behavior-and-communication/dos-and-donts-communicating-person-who-has
   Accessed on 01/08/2024

[468] Loef, M., & Walach, H. (2012). Fruit, vegetables and prevention of cognitive decline or dementia: A systematic review of cohort studies. *The Journal of Nutrition Health & Aging*, 16(7), 626–630. https://doi.org/10.1007/s12603-012-0097-x

[469] Jiang, X., Huang, J., Song, D., Deng, R., Wei, J., & Zhang, Z. (2017). Increased consumption of fruit and vegetables is related to a reduced risk of cognitive impairment and dementia: Meta-Analysis. *Frontiers in Aging Neuroscience*, 9, 18. https://doi.org/10.3389/fnagi.2017.00018

[470] Yaffe, K., Kanaya, A. M., Lindquist, K., Simonsick, E. M., Harris, T. B., Shorr, R. I., . . . Newman, A. B. (2004). The metabolic syndrome, inflammation, and risk of cognitive decline. *JAMA*, 292(18), 2237. https://doi.org/10.1001/jama.292.18.2237

[471] Charisis, S., Ntanasi, E., Yannakoulia, M., Anastasiou, C. A., Kosmidis, M. H., Dardiotis, E., . . . Scarmeas, N. (2021). Diet inflammatory index and dementia incidence. *Neurology*, 97(24). https://doi.org/10.1212/wnl.0000000000012973

[472] Cholerton, B., Baker, L. D., & Craft, S. (2013). Insulin, cognition, and dementia. *European Journal of Pharmacology*, 719(1–3), 170–179. https://doi.org/10.1016/j.ejphar.2013.08.008

[473] Joly-Amado, A., Gratuze, M., Benderradji, H., Vieau, D., Buée, L., & Blum, D. (2018). Relation mutuelle entre Tau et

signalisation centrale de l'insuline. *M S-medecine Sciences*, 34(11), 929–935. https://doi.org/10.1051/medsci/2018238

[474] Ornish, D., Madison, C., Kivipelto, M., Kemp, C., McCulloch, C. E., Galasko, D., Artz, J., Rentz, D., Lin, J., Norman, K., Ornish, A., Tranter, S., DeLamarter, N., Wingers, N., Richling, C., Kaddurah-Daouk, R., Knight, R., McDonald, D., Patel, L., Verdin, E., … Arnold, S. E. (2024). Effects of intensive lifestyle changes on the progression of mild cognitive impairment or early dementia due to Alzheimer's disease: a randomized, controlled clinical trial. *Alzheimer's research & therapy*, 16(1), 122. https://doi.org/10.1186/s13195-024-01482-z

[475] National Institute of Aging. (n.d.). Vascular Dementia: Causes, Symptoms, and Treatments. Retrieved from https://www.nia.nih.gov/health/vascular-dementia/vascular-dementia-causes-symptoms-and-treatments

[476] Lee, A. Y. (2011). Vascular dementia. *Chonnam Medical Journal*, 47(2), 66. https://doi.org/10.4068/cmj.2011.47.2.66

[477] Román, G. C. (2002). Vascular dementia may be the most common form of dementia in the elderly. *Journal of the Neurological Sciences*, 203–204, 7–10. https://doi.org/10.1016/s0022-510x(02)00252-6

[478] Perez, L., Helm, L., Sherzai, A., & Jaceldo-Siegl, K. (2012). Nutrition and vascular dementia. *The Journal of Nutrition Health & Aging*, 16(4), 319–324. https://doi.org/10.1007/s12603-012-0042-z

[479] Greenwood, C. E., & Parrott, M. D. (2016). Nutrition as a component of dementia risk reduction strategies. *Healthcare Management Forum*, 30(1), 40–45. https://doi.org/10.1177/0840470416662885

[480] Hughes, T. F., Andel, R., Small, B. J., Borenstein, A. R., Mortimer, J. A., Wolk, A., . . . Gatz, M. (2010). Midlife fruit and vegetable consumption and risk of dementia in later life in

Swedish twins. *The American Journal of Geriatric Psychiatry*, 18(5), 413–420. https://doi.org/10.1097/jgp.0b013e3181c65250

[481] Berding, K., Carbia, C., & Cryan, J. F. (2021). Going with the grain: Fiber, cognition, and the microbiota-gut-brain-axis. *Experimental Biology and Medicine*, 246(7), 796–811. https://doi.org/10.1177/1535370221995785

[482] Prokopidis, K., Giannos, P., Ispoglou, T., Witard, O. C., & Isanejad, M. (2022). Dietary Fiber Intake is Associated with Cognitive Function in Older Adults: Data from the National Health and Nutrition Examination Survey. *The American Journal of Medicine*, 135(8), e257–e262. https://doi.org/10.1016/j.amjmed.2022.03.022

[483] National Institute on Aging. (n.d.-a). Beyond the brain: The gut microbiome and Alzheimer's disease. Retrieved January 8, 2024, from https://www.nia.nih.gov/news/beyond-brain-gut-microbiome-and-alzheimers-disease Accessed on 01/08/2024.

[484] Yamagishi, K., Maruyama, K., Ikeda, A., Nagao, M., Noda, H., Umesawa, M., . . . Iso, H. (2022). Dietary fiber intake and risk of incident disabling dementia: the Circulatory Risk in Communities Study. *Nutritional Neuroscience*, 26(2), 148–155. https://doi.org/10.1080/1028415x.2022.2027592

[485] Barberger-Gateau, P., Raffaitin, C., Letenneur, L., Berr, C., Tzourio, C., Dartigues, J., & Alpérovitch, A. (2007). Dietary patterns and risk of dementia. *Neurology,* 69(20), 1921–1930. https://doi.org/10.1212/01.wnl.0000278116.37320.52

[486] Liu, X., Yan, Y., Li, F., & Zhang, D. (2016). Fruit and vegetable consumption and the risk of depression: A meta-analysis. *Nutrition*, 32(3), 296–302. https://doi.org/10.1016/j.nut.2015.09.009

[487] Bear, T., Dalziel, J. E., Coad, J., Roy, N. C., Butts, C. A., & Gopal, P. K. (2020). The role of the gut microbiota in dietary

interventions for depression and anxiety. *Advances in Nutrition*, 11(4), 890–907. https://doi.org/10.1093/advances/nmaa016

[488] Van Horn, J., Mayer, D., Chen, S., & Mayer, E. A. (2022). Role of diet and its effects on the gut microbiome in the pathophysiology of mental disorders. *Translational Psychiatry*, 12(1). https://doi.org/10.1038/s41398-022-01922-0

[489] Firth, J., Gangwisch, J. E., Borisini, A., Wootton, R. E., & Mayer, E. A. (2020). Food and mood: how do diet and nutrition affect mental wellbeing? *The BMJ*, m2382. https://doi.org/10.1136/bmj.m2382

[490] Adan, R. A., Van Der Beek, E. M., Buitelaar, J. K., Cryan, J. F., Hebebrand, J., Higgs, S., . . . Dickson, S. L. (2019). Nutritional psychiatry: Towards improving mental health by what you eat. *European Neuropsychopharmacology*, 29(12), 1321–1332. https://doi.org/10.1016/j.euroneuro.2019.10.011

[491] Yano, J. M., Yu, K., Donaldson, G. P., Shastri, G. G., Ann, P., Ma, L., . . . Hsiao, E. Y. (2015). Indigenous Bacteria from the Gut Microbiota Regulate Host Serotonin Biosynthesis. *Cell,* 161(2), 264–276. https://doi.org/10.1016/j.cell.2015.02.047

[492] Reigstad, C. S., Salmonson, C. E., Rainey, J. F., Szurszewski, J. H., Linden, D. R., Sonnenburg, J. L., . . . Kashyap, P. C. (2014). Gut microbes promote colonic serotonin production through an effect of short-chain fatty acids on enterochromaffin cells. *The FASEB Journal*, 29(4), 1395–1403. https://doi.org/10.1096/fj.14-259598

[493] Evrensel, A., & Ceylan, M. E. (2015). The Gut-Brain axis: the missing link in depression. *Clinical Psychopharmacology and Neuroscience : The Official Scientific Journal of the Korean College of Neuropsychopharmacology,* 13(3), 239–244. https://doi.org/10.9758/cpn.2015.13.3.239

[494] Saghafian, F., Malmir, H., Saneei, P., Milajerdi, A., Larijani, B., & Esmaillzadeh, A. (2018). Fruit and vegetable consumption and risk of depression: accumulative evidence from an updated

systematic review and meta-analysis of epidemiological studies. *British Journal of Nutrition*, 119(10), 1087–1101. https://doi.org/10.1017/s0007114518000697

[495] Kris-Etherton, P. M., Petersen, K. S., Hibbeln, J. R., Hurley, D. L., Kolick, V., Peoples, S., . . . Woodward-Lopez, G. (2020). Nutrition and behavioral health disorders: depression and anxiety. *Nutrition Reviews*, 79(3), 247–260. https://doi.org/10.1093/nutrit/nuaa025

[496] Aucoin, M., LaChance, L., Naidoo, U., Remy, D., Shekdar, T., Sayar, N., . . . Cooley, K. (2021). Diet and Anxiety: A scoping review. *Nutrients*, 13(12), 4418. https://doi.org/10.3390/nu13124418

[497] Głąbska, D., Guzek, D., Groele, B., & Gutkowska, K. (2020). Fruit and Vegetable Intake and Mental Health in Adults: A Systematic review. *Nutrients*, 12(1), 115. https://doi.org/10.3390/nu12010115

CHAPTER 10. PRECIOUS MIRACLE: PREGNANCY

[498] Lynch, C., Sundaram, R., Maisog, J. M., Sweeney, A., & Louis, G. M. B. (2014). Preconception stress increases the risk of infertility: results from a couple-based prospective cohort study—the LIFE study. *Human Reproduction*, 29(5), 1067–1075. https://doi.org/10.1093/humrep/deu032

[499] Grossman, P., Niemann, L., Schmidt, S., & Walach, H. (2004). Mindfulness-based stress reduction and health benefits. *Journal of Psychosomatic Research*, 57(1), 35–43. https://doi.org/10.1016/s0022-3999(03)00573-7

[500] Warriner, S., Crane, C., Dymond, M., & Krusche, A. (2018). An evaluation of mindfulness-based childbirth and parenting courses for pregnant women and prospective fathers/partners

within the UK NHS (MBCP-4-NHS). *Midwifery*, 64, 1–10. https://doi.org/10.1016/j.midw.2018.05.004

[501] Lönnberg, G., Jonas, W., Unternäehrer, E., Bränström, R., Nissen, E., & Niemi, M. (2020). Effects of a mindfulness based childbirth and parenting program on pregnant women's perceived stress and risk of perinatal depression–Results from a randomized controlled trial. *Journal of Affective Disorders*, 262, 133–142. https://doi.org/10.1016/j.jad.2019.10.048

[502] Veringa, I. K., De Bruin, E. I., Bardacke, N., Duncan, L. G., Van Steensel, F. J. A., Dirksen, C. D., & Bögels, S. M. (2016). 'I've Changed My Mind', Mindfulness-Based Childbirth and Parenting (MBCP) for pregnant women with a high level of fear of childbirth and their partners: study protocol of the quasi-experimental controlled trial. BMC Psychiatry, 16(1). https://doi.org/10.1186/s12888-016-1070-8

[503] Simionescu, G., Doroftei, B., Maftei, R., Obreja, B., Anton, E., Grab, D., ... Anton, C. (2021). The complex relationship between infertility and psychological distress (Review). *Experimental and Therapeutic Medicine*, 21(4). https://doi.org/10.3892/etm.2021.9737

[504] Craig, W. J., Mangels, A. R., Fresán, U., Marsh, K., Miles, F. L., Saunders, A., ... Orlich, M. J. (2021). The Safe and Effective Use of Plant-Based Diets with Guidelines for Health Professionals. *Nutrients*, 13(11), 4144. https://doi.org/10.3390/nu13114144

[505] Herrmann, K., Cano, S., Elío, I., Vergara, M. M., Giampieri, F., & Battino, M. (2015). Plant-Based and Plant-Rich Diet Patterns during Gestation: Beneficial Effects and Possible Shortcomings. *Advances in Nutrition*, 6(5), 581–591. https://doi.org/10.3945/an.115.009126

[506] Melina, V., Craig, W. J., & Levin, S. (2016). Position of the Academy of Nutrition and Dietetics: Vegetarian Diets. *Journal of the Academy of Nutrition and Dietetics*, 116(12), 1970–1980. https://doi.org/10.1016/j.jand.2016.09.025

[507] Sebastiani, G., Barbero, A. H., Borràs-Novell, C., Casanovà, M. A., Aldecoa-Bilbao, V., Andreu-Férnández, V., . . . García-Algar, Ó. (2019). The Effects of Vegetarian and Vegan Diet during Pregnancy on the Health of Mothers and Offspring. *Nutrients*, 11(3), 557. https://doi.org/10.3390/nu11030557

[508] Perry, A. R., Stephanou, A., & Rayman, M. P. (2022). Dietary factors that affect the risk of pre-eclampsia. *BMJ Nutrition, Prevention & Health*, 5(1), 118–133. https://doi.org/10.1136/bmjnph-2021-000399

[509] Esquivel, M. (2022). Nutritional status and nutrients related to Pre-Eclampsia risk. *American Journal of Lifestyle Medicine*, 17(1), 41–45. https://doi.org/10.1177/15598276221129841

[510] Streuling, I., Beyerlein, A., Rosenfeld, E., Schukat, B., & Von Kries, R. (2011). Weight gain and dietary intake during pregnancy in industrialized countries – a systematic review of observational studies. *Journal of Perinatal Medicine*, 39(2). https://doi.org/10.1515/jpm.2010.127

[511] Tomé-Carneiro, J., & Visioli, F. (2023). Plant-Based diets Reduce blood Pressure: A Systematic Review of Recent evidence. *Current Hypertension Reports*, 25(7), 127–150. https://doi.org/10.1007/s11906-023-01243-7

[512] Lee, K. W., Loh, H., Ching, S. M., Devaraj, N. K., & Hoo, F. K. (2020). Effects of Vegetarian Diets on Blood Pressure Lowering: A Systematic Review with Meta-Analysis and Trial Sequential Analysis. *Nutrients*, 12(6), 1604. https://doi.org/10.3390/nu12061604

[513] Del Re, A., & Aspry, K. (2022). Update on Plant-Based diets and cardiometabolic risk. *Current Atherosclerosis Reports*, 24(3), 173–183. https://doi.org/10.1007/s11883-022-00981-4

[514] Thomas, M., Calle, M. C., & Fernández, M. L. (2023). Healthy plant-based diets improve dyslipidemias, insulin resistance, and inflammation in metabolic syndrome. A narrative review.

Advances in Nutrition, 14(1), 44–54. https://doi.org/10.1016/j.advnut.2022.10.002

[515] Najjar, R., Moore, C. E., & Montgomery, B. D. (2018). A defined, plant-based diet utilized in an outpatient cardiovascular clinic effectively treats hypercholesterolemia and hypertension and reduces medications. *Clinical Cardiology*, 41(3), 307–313. https://doi.org/10.1002/clc.22863

[516] Yisahak, S. F., Hinkle, S., Mumford, S., Li, M., Andriessen, V. C., Grantz, K. L., . . . Grewal, J. (2020). Vegetarian diets during pregnancy, and maternal and neonatal outcomes. *International Journal of Epidemiology*, 50(1), 165–178. https://doi.org/10.1093/ije/dyaa200

[517] Kesary, Y., Avital, K., & Hiersch, L. (2020). Maternal plant-based diet during gestation and pregnancy outcomes. *Archives of Gynecology and Obstetrics*, 302(4), 887–898. https://doi.org/10.1007/s00404-020-05689-x

[518] Chen, Z., Qian, F., Liu, G., Li, M., Voortman, T., Tobias, D. K., . . . Zhang, C. (2021). Prepregnancy plant-based diets and the risk of gestational diabetes mellitus: a prospective cohort study of 14,926 women. *The American Journal of Clinical Nutrition*, 114(6), 1997–2005. https://doi.org/10.1093/ajcn/nqab275

[519] Schiattarella, A., Lombardo, M., Morlando, M., & Rizzo, G. (2021). The Impact of a Plant-Based Diet on Gestational Diabetes: A review. Antioxidants, 10(4), 557. https://doi.org/10.3390/antiox10040557

[520] Lambert, V., Muñoz, S. E., Gil, C., & Román, M. D. (2023). Maternal dietary components in the development of gestational diabetes mellitus: a systematic review of observational studies to timely promotion of health. *Nutrition Journal*, 22(1). https://doi.org/10.1186/s12937-023-00846-9

[521] Zhang, C., Liu, S., Solomon, C. G., & Hu, F. B. (2006). Dietary fiber intake, dietary glycemic load, and the risk for gestational

diabetes mellitus. *Diabetes Care,* 29(10), 2223–2230. https://doi.org/10.2337/dc06-0266

[522] Ötleş, S., & Özgöz, S. (2014). Health effects of dietary fiber. *Acta Scientiarum Polonorum,* 13(2), 191–202. https://doi.org/10.17306/j.afs.2014.2.8

[523] Veronese, N., Solmi, M., Caruso, M. G., Giannelli, G., Osella, A. R., Evangelou, E., . . . Tzoulaki, I. (2018). Dietary fiber and health outcomes: an umbrella review of systematic reviews and meta-analyses. *The American Journal of Clinical Nutrition,* 107(3), 436–444. https://doi.org/10.1093/ajcn/nqx082

[524] Mikkelsen, T. B., Østerdal, M. L., Knudsen, V. K., Haugen, M., Meltzer, H. M., Bakketeig, L. S., & Olsen, S. F. (2008). Association between a Mediterranean-type diet and risk of preterm birth among Danish women: a prospective cohort study. *Acta Obstetricia Et Gynecologica Scandinavica,* 87(3), 325–330. https://doi.org/10.1080/00016340801899347

[525] Barrett, J. R. (2013). Prenatal protection: Maternal diet may modify impact of PAHs. Environmental Health Perspectives, 121(10). https://doi.org/10.1289/ehp.121-a311

[526] Pedersen, M., Schoket, B., Godschalk, R., Wright, J., Von Stedingk, H., Törnqvist, M., . . . Kogevinas, M. (2013). Bulky DNA adducts in cord blood, maternal Fruit-and-Vegetable consumption, and birth weight in a European Mother–Child study (NewGeneris). *Environmental Health Perspectives,* 121(10), 1200–1206. https://doi.org/10.1289/ehp.120633

[527] Dietrich, M., Block, G., Pogoda, J. M., Buffler, P. A., Hecht, S. S., & Preston-Martin, S. (2005). A review: dietary and endogenously formed N-nitroso compounds and risk of childhood brain tumors. *Cancer Causes & Control,* 16(6), 619–635. https://doi.org/10.1007/s10552-005-0168-y

[528] Cleveland Clinic. (2023, November 16). Nitrates and nitrites: What are they and what foods have them? Retrieved from https://health.clevelandclinic.org/what-are-nitrates

[529] Pogoda, J. M., Preston-Martin, S., Howe, G. R., Lubin, F., Mueller, B. A., Holly, E. A., . . . Choi, W. (2009). An International Case-Control Study of Maternal Diet during Pregnancy and Childhood brain tumor Risk: A Histology-Specific Analysis by Food Group. *Annals of Epidemiology*, 19(3), 148–160. https://doi.org/10.1016/j.annepidem.2008.12.011

[530] Kominiarek, M. A., & Rajan, P. (2016). Nutrition recommendations in pregnancy and lactation. *Medical Clinics of North America*, 100(6), 1199–1215. https://doi.org/10.1016/j.mcna.2016.06.004

[531] Mullins, A., & Arjmandi, B. H. (2021b). Health benefits of Plant-Based Nutrition: Focus on beans in cardiometabolic diseases. *Nutrients,* 13(2), 519. https://doi.org/10.3390/nu13020519

[532] Wikipedia contributors. (2023a, December 10). Vigna mungo. Retrieved from https://en.wikipedia.org/wiki/Vigna_mungo

[533] Viswanathan, M. (2023b, August 1). Folic acid supplementation to prevent neural tube defects: A limited systematic review update for the U.S. Preventive Services Task Force. Retrieved from https://www.ncbi.nlm.nih.gov/books/NBK593614/

Made in the USA
Middletown, DE
19 September 2025